Coping With Celiac
the great masquerader

by
Aileen Bennett

A & G Publishing
Gulfport, MS 39507

To: Carol,
Best Wishes,
Aileen M. Bennett

DISCLAIMER
Any medical information contained in this book should not be considered as medical advice, nor should the information be used by individuals as such. Your doctor should be consulted for any opinion, diagnosis, or treatment in the matter of your health. Any treatment, medication, vitamin or supplement should not be initiated or undertaken without a doctor's authorization and supervision.

A & G Publishing
2907 Palmer Dr.
Gulfport, MS 39507

Library of Congress number: 98-93282

ISBN number: 0-9665353-0-8

Printed in United States of America
Cover design by Dolphin Press
Long Beach, MS

CONTENTS

**My thanks to Dr. Karen Wasserman
for the inspiration
and to Betty Malone
for the advice.**

Comments

"Aileen Bennett's writing on the personal stories of individuals diagnosed with celiac sprue is a must-read for anyone diagnosed with the disease. The book features the patient's perspective on the disease. Each individual's experience is unique and highly informative. This book clearly illustrates the many faces of celiac sprue. Thankfully, it offers a refreshing dose of humanity to the medical literature on celiac sprue."
John D. MCKee, M.D.

***

"As a registered dietitian my interaction with the celiacs in our support group on the coast has been an educational experience. I am much more aware of the day to day problems the celiac encounters and I have gained invaluable information and insight from them. The celiac patient who follows the gluten-free diet knows the diet better than the average dietitian who encounters it occasionally. The best resource for the new celiac after an initial diet instruction by a registered dietitian is an old compliant celiac. Our support group offers members the opportunity to meet and interact with other celiacs."
Annette

***

1

THE COVER

The cover has a lot of symbolism: the center circle represents the mind, the next circle represents celiac and the box represents the body.

Starting at the center circle (the mind), red represents the turmoil before diagnosis, the gray shaded down to black ,represents the relief and then calmness after diagnosis.

In the next circle (celiac) the black represents celiac in its dark rage tormenting the body; gray is celiac when it is dormant, but still lurking in the shadows and white represents celiac under control.

In the square (the body) red represents the pain of celiac when it is active; gray represents the mystery of celiac when it is dormant and black represents the calmness when celiac is under control.

INTRODUCTION

This book is about sharing: shared stories, recipes, information about books that have been of help, and general advice. Hopefully, all of this coming together will be of some help to future and present celiac victims. I hope that the facts in the following stories will open the eyes of people without celiac disease as to what the disorder is all about. Everyone who has contributed to the contents of this book seems to have the same point of view. They want to help each other, which is a very basic element to a successful approach to deal with their every day problems. This is only a small step in the right direction that will lead to better understanding of the disorder. Understanding leads to harmony and harmony can only bring about good things to all of us.

The purpose of this book is to inform the public of the problems that celiacs face everyday. Every meal is a challenging mental experience and we must determine what is in every mouthful of food before we eat it. Re-education in this category is a must. Some foods may contain ingredients which, in turn, may have a small amount of gluten. Example: modified food starch or natural flavorings must be avoided because their origination is questionable. In one story caramel flavoring was a problem.

Some celiacs go for years and years with elusive symptoms that sometimes add up to a puzzling situation. Celiac disease has a maze of symptoms and every case of celiac seems to be different. This book will demonstrate these circumstances with twenty compelling stories from celiacs. Hopefully you will get a clearer picture of the problems they face everyday, before diagnosis and after diagnosis. The following stories are true. Many of the same problems arise; the most common being the lack of a timely diagnosis and a scarcity of information for the newly-diagnosed celiac.

The standard of a firm diagnosis is a biopsy of the small intestine, but in some of the following stories the participants stumbled across their diagnosis by unconventional means. I hope that you will understand that in these cases, after years of suffering, the participants were overwhelmed by their symptoms which made them very vulnerable. Therefore, they were willing to grasp at any possible solution that was offered. Then, the thought of going through a gluten challenge to confirm a diagnosis seemed to be too devastating for them. In each case the doctor agreed with their decision to forego the gluten challenge. These unusual cases help define that more research is needed to prove that standardized testing should be implemented, so patients will not have to sort through their unusual symptoms alone.

The first Chapter is a technical definition of celiac disease, but hang in there; the stories are quite interesting.

A joy shared is doubled, and a sorrow shared is halved. (Author unknown.)

WHAT IS CELIAC?

Celiac disease, also known as sprue, is sometimes hard to diagnose as was my case which will attest to this statement. After 58 years of maladies of unexplained origin which included bouts of diarrhea, anemia, muscle wasting, hair loss, and general fatigue, a diagnosis was made after a prolonged bout of diarrhea which resulted in my losing about 20 pounds. The doctor then told me to avoid gluten. This sounds simple enough, but following his advice was not easy. Celiac is a complicated disease which takes a convoluted path through your body with devastating results.

The following definition is quite technical and it has a lot of important words that celiacs hear over and over--plus a few that may be unfamiliar. A glossary is provided in the back of the book; the words contained in the glossary are italicized. With this information a celiac will be better informed; they will more fully understand their situation and will be better equipped to ask sensible questions with a broader understanding of the disease.

According to The Merck Manual of Diagnosis and Therapy the definition of celiac disease is as follows:

"A chronic intestinal malabsorption disorder caused by intolerance to gluten, characterized by a flat *jejunal mucosa* with clinical and/or histology improvement following withdrawal of dietary gluten."

"This hereditary disorder is caused by sensitivity to *gliadin* fraction of *gluten*, a cereal protein found in wheat and rye and to a lesser degree in barley and oats. *Gliadin*, acting as *antigen*, combines with *antibodies* to form an immune complex in the intestinal *mucosa* that promotes the aggregation of K (killer*) lymphocytes*. In some way these lymphocytes cause mucosal damage with loss of *villi* and proliferation of *crypt cells*. The prevalence of celiac disease

5

varies from about 1:300 in southwest Ireland to 1:5000 or more in North America. There is no single genetic marker."

"Celiac disease may be *symptomatic* or *asymptomatic* and present at any age, often without diarrhea or *steatorrhea*. Primary symptoms and signs may be short stature, infertility, *anemia*, recurrent *aphthous stomatis*, or *dermatitis herpetiformis*."

"Family studies show that typical *mucosal* abnormalities appear in apparently healthy siblings of affected patients. The disease may present itself for the first time in infancy or adulthood, but it should not be assumed that an adult presentation is the first manifestation. Although the patient may have no knowledge of childhood disease, his mother may recall abdominal symptoms. If the adult patient is significantly smaller than his siblings and has evidence of mild bowing deformities of the long bones, the likelihood of latent or undiagnosed childhood disease is increased."

"In infancy, symptoms are absent until the child eats food containing gluten. The child fails to thrive, begins to pass pale, malodorous, bulky stools, and suffers painful abdominal bloating. Iron deficiency anemia develops and, if *hypoproteinemia* is severe enough, *edema* appears. Celiac disease is strongly suspected in a pale, *querulous* child, with wasted buttocks and a pot belly, who has an adequate diet. (thus ruling out protein-calorie malnutrition.)"

"In adults, celiac disease is usually diagnosed when malabsorption is found in conjunction with a flat *jejunal biopsy* not due to some recognizable cause and gluten is shown to be of *etiologic* significance. Family incidence is a valuable clue. It may present, apparently for the first time, at any age. The average age of presentation in women is 10 to 15 years earlier than in men, because *amenorrhea* or *anemia* in pregnancy may heighten clinical suspicion."

"There is no single presentation. Many symptoms (eg. anemia, weight loss, bone pain, *paresthesia, edema*, and skin disorders) also occur, the real diagnosis is unlikely to be missed. Without direct clues, malabsorption may not be suspected. There tends to be iron-deficiency in children and *folate* deficiency *anemia* in adults."

"Diagnosis is suspected on the basis of the symptoms and signs, enhanced by laboratory and x-ray studies, and confirmed by biopsy showing a flat *mucosa* and a clinical and *histologic* improvement on a gluten-free diet. *Jejunal biopsy* can be performed even in small infants, but to obviate the risk of bowel perforation, only an experienced investigator should do the test. If a biopsy cannot be done, the diagnosis may have to depend on the clinical and laboratory response to a *gluten*-free diet."

"While *gluten* withdrawal has transformed the prognosis for children and substantially improved it for adults, there is still some mortality from the disease, mainly among adults whose condition is severe from the beginning. An important cause of death is the development of lymphoreticular disease (especially intestinal *lymphoma*). It is not known whether this risk is diminished by scrupulous adherence to *gluten*-free diet. Some patients can tolerate the reintroduction of *gluten* into the diet. It is not certain whether this means that some mild cases can achieve complete remission (unlikely) or whether the *gluten* toxicity is a nonspecific effect on a *mucosa* previously damaged by an acute bacterial or viral *enteritis*. In any case, apparent clinical remission is often associated with *histologic* relapse that is detected only if review biopsies are performed."

"**Dietary gluten must be excluded:** Ingesting even small amounts may prevent remission or induce relapse. *Gluten* is so widely used (eg., in commercial soups, sauces, ice creams, hot dogs) that patients need detailed lists of foodstuffs to avoid and expert advice from a dietitian familiar with the problems of celiac disease."

7

"Supplementary vitamins, minerals, and *hematinics* may be given, depending on the degree of deficiency. In mild cases no supplementation may be necessary. In severe cases comprehensive replacement may be required. Sometimes children (but rarely) adults who are seriously ill on first diagnosis may require a period of IV feeding."

"A few patients respond poorly or not at all to gluten withdrawal, because the diagnosis is incorrect or because the disease has entered a *refractory* phase."[1]

---

[1]From: The Merck Manual of Diagnosis and Therapy, Edition 16, pp.826-828, edited by Robert Berkow. Rahway, NJ; Merck & Co., Inc., copyright 1992.

Lucille

Lucille was born in Texas in the late 1920's, and has lived there ever since. She was diagnosed at a very young age with celiac disease and very little was known about the disorder. One of her doctors said, "The malady, almost unknown in this part of the country, is common in tropical climates and is a problem of malnutrition." Since the exact cause of the disease had not yet been discovered when Lucille was diagnosed, a trial and error diet method was used to try to control it. Most of Lucille's first six years was spent in and out of the hospital, mostly in.

The Great Depression was in full swing, food was scarce, and times were hard. Lucille remembers these times very vividly even though many, many years have passed.

She recalls some of her earliest childhood memories with ease. She says, "I remember always being hungry and I always cried for food. My father used to say my eyes were bigger than my stomach."

Lucille's father was not very tolerant of the toddler's plight. She says, "Once I was crying for more food and my father rubbed a whole plate of jelly in my face. The jelly burned my little eyes and I remember my mom pleading with him to stop it, that I was a sick child." Not knowing that the gluten in the food Lucille ingested was causing her symptoms, her father had mistakenly thought she was just being a naughty child. She reflects, "This was very cruel as I was getting no nutrients from my food and that was the reason I was always starving."

When Lucille was about four years old she remembers being so hungry that she would wander the neighborhood and rummage through garbage cans looking for scraps of food. She says, "I'd go to a neighbor's and steal left over cornbread out of the garbage, and get deathly sick and my mother would know I had been stealing food."

Some people add wheat flour to their cornmeal when making cornbread. Evidently the neighbor did this; otherwise, Lucille should have able to tolerate the cornbread.

Lucille recalls several events that happened during one hospital stay that lasted for several years. The doctors wanted to do exploratory surgery; they told her mother that her stomach and intestines were in nine knots, but the surgery was never performed. The other traumatic incident happened at about five years of age; she remembers waking up in the middle of the night floating in excrement. She says, "The nurse got mad and put me back in baby diapers. I cried until two a.m., because I was so humiliated. About three a.m. they called my mom and she sent my dad to the hospital. He came there drunk with another strange woman. I'd never seen her before and my dad told me that she was my new mother. I didn't understand and kept crying until the hospital called my mom and told her what my dad had done. So, all 300 pounds of her had to come to the hospital to quiet me down; this was about four a.m. I finally quieted down after I realized I still had my mom." These were just some of the horrors that she, as a celiac, had to face back then. Not even the nurse had compassion.

Lucille's many hospital stays finally came to an end and she was at home all the time, but because she had spent so much time in the hospital she was a stranger in her own home. Lucille's brothers and sisters hardly knew her; they had not bonded due to their frequent and prolonged separations.

Food was still scarce, and what was available was modest fare which included a lot of soup and bread, but very little meat, few vegetables and fruit. However, Lucille received special food: bananas, jello, limburger cheese and dried chicken gizzards. (Yes dried.) The other children were very jealous of the attention that Lucille received from their mother and was treated as an outsider by them. The other children did not care about the limburger cheese and chicken gizzards, but they longed for some of the jello and bananas that Lucille ate almost every day. And, the irony of it all is that Lucille was yearning for some of the food that her brothers and sisters could eat. She just wanted to be "normal." Of course, the family did not know the gravity of Lucille's disorder. It was especially hard for the other children to realize that Lucille was even sick; she looked very normal to them.

Because of the malnutrition caused by celiac, Lucille was always exceptionally thin. The other kids liked to torment her, especially her brother. He would taunt Lucille by calling her "bird legs." Her mother would try to smooth things over by telling her son to hush. This was usually met with the response of "tweetie, tweetie" by the boy as he ran away. These encounters made Lucille very sad, she felt as though she didn't belong anywhere; neither the stark environment of the hospital nor her life at home gave her any comfort. She says, " I just couldn't understand why my sisters and brothers hated me so much because I got jello and bananas. But, that's what kept me alive and my mother made sure I had some food. I love her for that."

Lucille, her brothers and sisters had a favorite spot to play, White Rock Lake in Dallas. She says, "I would eat the road gravel and dirt because my body was craving minerals. I didn't realize then, why I ate the gravel or dirt. I used to get spanked for this."

At the age of twelve or thirteen she seemed to be recovering; the doctors came to the conclusion that Lucille had grown out of celiac. Her mother was relieved to hear this. Lucille started to eat regular food again, but little did they know that Lucille still suffered from the malady; evidently, the celiac had only gone into a dormant stage. For the next sixty years, Lucille did not even think of celiac disease.

She married a kind and understanding man and had one daughter. At last, her life seemed to be normal. She now had a family where warmth and closeness prevailed. The affection and understanding that she lacked from her family in her childhood was now fulfilled by her own loving husband and child.

Fewer health problems plagued Lucille during these years; however, she did suffer from asthma and frequent colds. When these respiratory ailments would strike, they seemed to last longer for Lucille than most other people.

Recently, after experiencing some other health problems, Lucille was re-diagnosed with celiac disease. She says, "I thought I had outgrown celiac, but I have learned you never do. I feel sometimes that God watched over me and took care of me." Well, God certainly must have been watching over her because Lucille has now lived for more than seventy years even though the doctors predicted many years ago that she would not live past the age of twelve.

Still, she is not close to her brothers and sisters and has very little contact with them. She heard that one of her sisters recently died from diabetes at the age of sixty-four. Lucille will never know if her sister also had celiac disease.

Since gluten has been discovered to be the culprit in celiac disease, children and adults have a wider choice of food; no more dried chicken gizzards or Limburger cheese !!

ALEXANDRA

Alexandra resides in a beautiful area of the country, Louisiana, where living goes at a slow pace and food is generally the centerpiece of conversation. If you are a celiac and happen to live there, you have one up on the rest of us celiacs because red beans and rice is a favorite which is gluten-free. According to a Louisiana tradition of many years ago, red beans and rice was cooked on Monday which was wash day, and the water drained from the cooked rice was used to starch the clothes. Not only was your meal gluten-free, but your laundry was, too.

About two years ago Alexandra thought she had a bad case of the flu that would not go away, so she decided to go to the emergency weekend clinic where she was seen by the doctor of family medicine. When she related her symptoms to him he prescribed Metamucil which only made her condition worse. Her best friend, a doctor, recommended that Alexandra go to a gastroenterologist for a work-up and referred her to a specialist in Jefferson Parish (In Louisiana counties are referred to as Parishes.) For years, Alexandra had been taking iron pills which no longer seemed to help; her friend, the doctor, was aware of this fact and reminded Alexandra to tell the gastroenterologist.

Within a short time, Alexandra saw the specialist and based on the symptoms that she was experiencing the doctor was pretty sure that it was celiac. A biopsy was scheduled to be performed a short time later and the results confirmed the doctor's suspicion, a positive diagnosis of celiac.

The gastroenterologist was familiar with the disease which made the diagnosis easy and fast in Alexandra's case, but little information was available for her about the gluten-free diet. However, a friend who works at a local newspaper helped find some information in the food section of an old edition. The article contained a telephone number for a local support group which Alexandra contacted, but their contact person told Alexandra horrifying stories about celiac which was very different from what the doctor had told her; she quickly decided not to attend any meetings, but she did receive some updated material.

Alexandra's main support group is her friends and family. She says, "My sister and my best friend mailed me cookbooks (gluten free) and all those crazy flours we use. My room-mate looked up recipes on the Internet and became intrigued. We started experimenting with baking together and she discovered several great variations on cornbread. And my mom bought me a bread machine! So I did manage some great support."

Alexandra hopes that we can all learn a valuable lesson from her situation. She stresses that we should try and be aware that a newly diagnosed celiac is very vulnerable; emphasize what a celiac **can** eat, not what they cannot. This will point the newly diagnosed celiac in the right direction in a positive manner and will not cause them to turn away.

Alexandra's heritage is Scottish on her mother's side of the family and her father's side is Anglo, as well, which gives a big clue that celiac disease may be a problem in the family because it is more prevalent in that area of the world; also heredity plays a major role in its course in a person's life. She knows of no one else in her family that has been diagnosed with celiac, but she has her own suspicions about a couple of family members who have not been tested for the disease for various reasons.

"Living in New Orleans has actually helped me be gluten-free," states Alexandra, "because of the likelihood of entering a restaurant where a full time chef is very conscious of what is put into the food they prepare and a waitstaff who are required to know what they are serving, it is very beneficial and much easier than what other people are dealing with in other cities. Also, when frying seafood in the

South it is common to use fish fry (corn flour) or corn meal. So, I don't miss this very important food,"

With such marvelous foods that Louisiana has to offer you would only expect that Alexandra would have a delicious recipe which she is willing to share with us. Her favorite is Polenta pizza, a blend of healthful, fresh vegetables with a tasty cornbread crust that melts in your mouth. This recipe is filling and it certainly soothes your hunger pangs. Polenta pizza has several pluses. It will be a big hit with everyone, even your gluten-eating friends; you will want to make this recipe again and again because it is simple and you can add more of your favorite vegetables or other items. Most celiacs have become very creative when a good recipe is converted to gluten-free status and Alexandra has certainly done a good job with Polenta pizza.

Polenta Pizza

3/4 cups rice flour
1 1/4 cups cornmeal
2 teaspoons baking powder
1 teaspoon salt
1teaspoon xanthan gum or guar gum
1 egg
1cup milk
1/4 cup melted butter

Sift all dry ingredients. Beat egg; add milk and butter. Combine with dry ingredients and then spread into a sheet cake pan (9x13). Bake at 350 degrees for about 20 minutes.

Alexandra uses a red onion, a green and red bell pepper, a yellow squash and a zucchini for her toppings; use as much or as little as you like. Chop and sauté your favorite vegetables until tender. The onions should be clear. Spread over crust. Pour pasta sauce over the top (about 3/4 of a jar) and pile on the cheddar and mozzarella cheese.

Put it back in the oven for about 15 minutes· until everything is hot and the cheese is melted. Don't leave it in the oven too long as the crust will get mushy.

You will certainly enjoy this dish because the cornbread crust has a hearty taste and you and your friends will like it better than regular pizza as a welcome change of pace.

RUTH

Ruth was a happy, curly headed child. She was chubby, which is unusual for a celiac and showed no symptoms at this early age. Despite the fact that at the age of six Ruth became very cranky, lost a lot of weight, and her hair straightened out she was a very healthy child. In fact, her siblings had a number of childhood diseases which included chicken pox, mumps and measles, but she had only one, chicken pox. Ruth's mother taught kindergarten in her home; although the students had a number of colds and the usual childhood diseases, Ruth never contracted any of them. She recalls, "I was very, very healthy, and I did not ever even have a cold until I was in college." She did have a big problem with her teeth; they always needed filling because they were very soft and her fingernails would break very easily. These symptoms, she later found out, were an indication of a lack of nutrients.

At 40 years of age Ruth had a hysterectomy because she suffered from fibroids. Also, she began a long road to recovery from alcoholism; she had been drinking excessively for 20 years and has been in recovery for over 14 years now. Ruth states, "I tend to get the DON'T diseases: don't drink and don't eat wheat."

At 50 years of age Ruth married and moved from Ohio to North Carolina, a beautiful, mountainous region in the southwestern part of the state, where the leaves on the trees in the fall present a spectacular cloak of vibrant color. Even an accomplished artist could not outdo Mother Nature in her display of warm and brilliant hues.

Her new spouse loved wheat products, especially bagels which enticed Ruth to eat more of them. Her wheat intake tripled, at least, and she also included oatmeal for breakfast quite frequently. As a child Ruth did not particularly care for pasta and bread, but preferred corn, meat, vegetables, and especially potatoes which was one of her favorites.

Ruth's health began to deteriorate; the flu struck five or six times each year and chronic bronchitis developed into a lung problem. Ruth made an appointment with her general practitioner who referred her to a specialist in Knoxville, Tennessee. A number of tests were performed which revealed a spot on her lungs. The diagnosis was negative, but then she developed pneumonia and began to lose a lot of weight. Her average weight was 135 and she was 5' 8" tall. After losing down to 115 pounds severe depression set in, and Ruth became very irritable. She made another appointment with her general practitioner who prescribed an antidepressant. After having a severe reaction to the drug, the GP suggested that Ruth see a psychiatrist so that she could be monitored for a serotonin adjustment. The psychiatrist prescribed a milder antidepressant which made her ears ring terribly and her muscles twitch uncontrollably; she began to have severe muscle cramps in her legs. Intermittent diarrhea developed that lasted for months and was diagnosed as irritable bowel syndrome which was attributed to stress. Ruth's health steadily declined and the diarrhea persisted.

After several months her husband left and her photography business started to go downhill because she had gotten to the point that she was so weak she could not even carry her cameras. This made work very difficult. Her business further declined because she could not work regularly. Mouth sores and yeast infections began to be a problem and the ringing in her ears continued.

Doctors attributed the symptoms to a variety of things, mainly stress. Since her husband had left, she did not know how she was going to make a living; nothing was going well. Her husband began teaching at a university that was a two hour drive away. They have not spoken to each other for over a year now, so he is unaware that Ruth was diagnosed with celiac disease.

Ruth was scheduled for her yearly GYN exam and upon seeing the doctor she happened to mention the frequent bouts of diarrhea. He was very concerned and suggested that she get checked by a specialist. She told the GYN doctor that she had been diagnosed with irritable bowel syndrome and he suggested that she go to a surgeon for a colonscope. Feeling uncomfortable about going to a surgeon for a GI problem, she consulted her general practitioner for further advice and he referred her to a gastroenterologist. The diagnosis was, she recalls, the GERD and a heartburn medication was prescribed. The doctor thought she may also have ulcers or an ulcerated colon. A procedure was scheduled to check for this, but Ruth was unhappy with the doctor and did not go back. Instead she went back to her general practitioner for more advice, but got no satisfaction. The heartburn got worse, but the medication did help somewhat.

Deciding to take it upon herself to go to a nearby university medical center, she called the GI clinic and made an appointment with a gastroenterologist there. To Ruth's surprise, a diagnosis was made in about five minutes after she arrived in the office. When the doctor came in Ruth related her symptoms; he then described a very rare disorder known as celiac disease, explaining that she sure had the classic symptoms. He was very knowledgeable about the disorder and answered all her questions. A lot of blood work and a biopsy of her small intestines was ordered. The doctor was quite sure Ruth had the disease. His diagnosis was confirmed when the biopsy came back positive.

The doctor told Ruth that she had to adhere to a strict gluten-free diet the rest of her life. He then gave her a short explanation of the diet and scheduled her for an appointment with a dietitian for the following month. Ruth was very perplexed. What was gluten? Her stress increased because she was given very little information about the diet.

Ruth returned home; realizing she had no idea what was going on, immediately she called her friends asking them to get some information off the Internet. Even though Ruth's appointment was still a month away she called the dietitian explaining the situation. She said that a month was far too long for Ruth to wait to straighten her diet out and mailed Ruth a small pamphlet which was not very helpful. Thank goodness Ruth's friends came to the rescue. They accumulated enough information for her to start on the gluten-free diet right away.

Realizing that some of her symptoms were due to malabsorption caused by celiac disease, she started to take a lot of vitamins which included a liquid vitamin B that she thought would be more digestible. Ruth concluded that for years she had gotten very few nutrients from the food that she had eaten.

Finally, it was time for the scheduled appointment with dietitian who gave Ruth two more pamphlets and explained them for only a short time. Then the dietitian started to discuss hidden glutens with Ruth which was very fascinating; the discussion revealed some useful information. (Example: if a chute at a plant is dusted with a wheat flour to make the product flow better; the flour may not be listed in the ingredients and for some celiacs just this minor amount could be troublesome). Ruth then got her computer hooked up to the Internet so that she could search more diligently for information about celiac. She joined a celiac news group and a chat room which helped enormously. Ruth states "I keep tripping over gluten; yes." She continued to have about two bouts of diarrhea a week.

The photography business finally went under. Before being diagnosed she was so sick that when a client would call to make an appointment Ruth would hope that they would cancel and that attitude came across over the phone. Fewer and fewer appointments were made. Her energy was sapped and she had a hard time focusing the cameras because she could not function a good deal of the time; the portraits were simply not the quality they were before she became sick. Work dried up; she finally laid off her entire staff and she soon may be destitute. Ruth attributes her plight solely to celiac. The only up side to this was that she had more time to gather information about celiac. She plans to search for a job in the bigger cities nearby which provide more job opportunities.

Within three days of going on the gluten-free diet Ruth noticed quite a difference and felt much better. The depression lifted within a week, the irritability was gone and it only comes back when gluten is ingested. Within a day after ingesting gluten she becomes very, very irritable, but most of the time she feels like her normal self.

As a result of going on the gluten-free diet, Ruth gained about 20 pounds; her muscles returned and she even has a shape with a little rear end. Her skin no longer looks like it belongs to a crocodile or a 90 year old person; it is smooth and moist. Ruth states, "There is just a world of difference in my whole body. I did not realize how bad my memory had gotten." Looking back she can recall at least 15 symptoms which included going from room to room in a daze, not knowing what she was doing. She is still on antidepressants, but she has an appointment soon and the doctor is considering taking her off them as the symptoms of depression are gone. Her memory loss has also cleared up which proves that the gluten-free diet is certainly working.

Since Ruth received no information about support groups from either the doctor or the dietitian, the search was continued on the Internet where several were promptly located. She joined every organization in order to get their newsletters because she was desperate for more information.

21

Ruth's heritage is Irish and English; she knows of no one else in her family who has been diagnosed with celiac. In fact, no one in her family has ever heard of celiac. Ruth suspects that her older sister may be suffering from the disorder, although the sister's symptoms left several years ago. Her sister suffered form cracked skin and a rash on her back and elbows for most of her life. Ruth is going to try to talk her into being tested.

A plan to lobby for more research is an idea that Ruth thinks needs to be implemented on the grass roots level, and better food labeling needs to be addressed. Hopefully, the future for Ruth will be brighter, since she has conquered two debilitating disorders. With these adjustments in dietary habits her life will be fuller in the future.

Food and drink are the medicines that we take every day of our lives. (Author unknown)

LIZ

Liz was born in Ireland in 1955 and now resides in a quiet suburban area of Dublin, the Capitol of Ireland. Liz faired well as a baby, but as soon as solid food was introduced into her diet things went awry; every time she was fed she threw up. She had the classic symptoms of celiac: white, floating, smelly stools. She failed to thrive, and even lost a lot of weight. Her mother stated, "Liz finally just refused to eat solid food altogether as though she knew that food was making her sick." Her mother thought that her darling child was just going to fade away.

At about 18 months Liz was diagnosed with celiac disease, and after being put on the gluten-free diet, she thrived. Liz does not recall if a biopsy was performed or if the diagnosis was based on dietary trial and error.

At the age of seven, following the advice of the doctor, Liz came off the gluten-free diet. She seemed to have no more of the classic symptoms of the disease after gluten was introduced into her meals again. The celiac, evidently, had gone dormant. She had only the usual childhood diseases: chicken pox, measles, etc. Otherwise, Liz seemed to be quite healthy, although she was a bit thin and slightly underweight for her height.

Later, Liz started developing long-lasting colds that recurred frequently; she also began to have odd bouts of queasiness and gas. Her doctor seemed to be familiar with celiac disease when Liz mentioned her medical history, but the doctor did not suggest any attempt at re-diagnosis and no recommendation was made for Liz to resume the gluten-free diet. Instead, the doctor went along with the theory that Liz had "grown out of it."

In November of 1993, while traveling in Burma, Liz got, as she states, "one hell of a dose of gastroenteritis with fever, vomiting; watery, mucousy, uncontrollable diarrhea, the works." She was out of reach of medical help and the nearest facility was miles and miles away. She did the only thing that she could do; she treated herself with lots of fluids and a few Immodium tablets that were on hand. Liz stated, "I knew that if I had been able to seek medical help, I would have most likely been admitted to the hospital. I never got a diagnosis of dysentery per se, but I sure had something bad. I had the distinct feeling that my whole gut had been torn out of me and was being replaced. I can't describe it any better than that. It was a definite feeling that I had a whole new insides."

Liz slowly began to eat solid food again and after her travels she returned to Ireland. During the following year, she developed numerous respiratory infections and was then diagnosed with post-infectious asthma. She was very anemic, felt fatigued a lot of the time and was starting to have menopausal-like symptoms. When her respiratory physician reviewed her medical history, he referred her to a gastroenterologist. A short time later a biopsy was performed, and she was re-diagnosed, as she suspected, with celiac disease. She was promptly put on a gluten-free diet. After a short time all her symptoms began to subside and within a few months the symptoms cleared up all together.

Liz discussed the "trigger-factor" for the re-appearance of celiac (after 32 years of apparently no symptoms) with her gastroenterologist and he agreed that the gastro episode in Burma could have been the "trigger." He said that it is impossible to determine precisely what triggers any case of dormant celiac disease to start producing more overt symptoms. He explained that certain factors such as a severe gastro infection, like the one that she contracted in Burma, have been mentioned in quite a few cases. "I didn't ask for references, but I'm quite sure some of these cases are documented," says Liz.

The gastroenterologist did some blood tests, which indicated that some of her nutrient values were slightly low, but he felt that Liz would improve quickly just being on the gluten-free diet since they were not too terribly low. Liz felt fatigued and she was slightly anemic. The respiratory therapist, but not her general practitioner, recommended that Liz start taking vitamins.

Liz was referred to a dietitian, but since being on the diet as a child, she already knew a lot about it. The dietitian gave Liz a handbook from the Celiac Society of Ireland which she joined. She soon located a celiac news group (The List) on the Internet and subscribed. These two sources gave her more useful information than the dietitian did.

The gluten-free diet really helped. "It made all the difference in the world." stated Liz. One of Liz' cousins was diagnosed with celiac disease as a child and was on the gluten-free diet back then, but the disease, evidently, had gone into a dormant stage because she returned to a normal diet with no apparent symptoms of celiac afterwards. Liz has lost contact with this cousin, so she cannot discuss her re-diagnosis and suggests that she, too, should be checked again.

Liz found that the diet was very hard to deal with when she was first re-diagnosed as an adult after so many years of eating everything, but she has now devised lot of ways of coping. One thing that definitely helps is that she always keeps a good stock of gluten-free treats handy. One of the main regrets that Liz has about the gluten-free diet is, "I do miss being able to drink a pint of Guiness," she says in dismay.

Liz has a wonderful dish that will appeal to everyone, a version of Ratatouille with kidney beans.

Ratatouille

The proportions are variable, so just add a lot of what you like and just a little, or delete, the ingredients that you do not like.

Chop and sauté onions, garlic, courgette (zucchini), and mushrooms.

Add diced red and green bell peppers and one can of chopped tomatoes

Salt

Pepper

Chopped Basil (fresh, if available).

Cooked kidney beans

Heat through for about 10 to 15 minutes and serve with brown rice, millet or gluten free pasta.

This dish will especially appeal to vegetarians. An excellent main dish and easy to prepare, it is a good source of protein.

Beryl

Beryl lives in Canada and is mostly Irish, with a little English and Scottish somewhere in her background which puts her in a category to be a prime candidate for inheriting celiac disease.

As a child, Beryl was healthy even though she had foamy, floaty stools. Not realizing this was a problem, she never complained. No other celiac symptoms were present at this time; she was not emaciated which is a typical childhood symptom.

Beryl developed what she thought was a severe attack of stomach flu in December, 1995. This malady continued off and on until March, 1996. Not knowing what the underlying problem was, she excluded all meat, poultry, fish and other seafood because she could no longer digest them. Her diet then included a lot of bread and pasta, more like a vegetarian diet.

Her stomach problems continued into May. Beryl was plagued with extreme fatigue, diarrhea, gas and bloating, but quickly gained 44 pounds due to a compulsion to eat. Never satisfied, she had the feeling that she was getting very little nutrition from her food. She developed tingling in her extremities and her energy was completely sapped, all she wanted to do was sleep. She went from a regular regimen of lifting weights to not being able to climb a flight of stairs. Beryl developed brain fuzziness and was unable to concentrate on her daily tasks; then moodiness and depression crept into her life. The diarrhea developed into bloody stools filled with mucous and she started having problems with her menstrual cycle. However, she still did not lose any weight. This certainly sounds like celiac masquerading.

Beryl visited her general practitioner whose diagnosis was irritable bowel syndrome, but even after the diagnosis symptoms persisted. She started to do some research of her own. After posting her symptoms on the Internet, a return e-mail suggested that she read "The List" to see if it was relevant. Was it ever! She downloaded a lot of useful information, which included the gluten-free diet, and quickly decided to try the diet just to see if it would affect her. A remarkable difference was noticed. She felt much better.

Immediately, a request was made to her general practitioner for a referral to see a gastroenterologist. An appointment was scheduled for October, 1996 almost a year after the symptoms had begun. When Beryl saw the specialist, he diagnosed her with hemorrhoids and postviral fatigue syndrome without doing any tests. He concluded that since she was not thin it was impossible for her to have celiac. (She had actually gained weight.) He was, however, familiar with the classic symptoms of the disease and an adult who had gained weight, with diarrhea, did not fit into this category. This conclusion seems logical. The doctor was very convincing and Beryl, thinking her problems were now solved, strayed from the gluten-free diet.

Symptoms persisted, which convinced her that the diagnosis was not correct. In April, 1997 she requested another referral to a second gastroenterologist, who happened to be very familiar with the disorder. He proceeded with an interview, blood screening, and biopsy which proved she certainly did have celiac disease. However, he was still puzzled by Beryl's symptoms of weight gain, brain fuzziness and lack of concentration, but he was willing to do some research on her behalf.

Because the doctor was quite knowledgeable about celiac, he answered all her questions and explained about malabsorption. Her blood work showed that she was in the normal range. Information was given to her about the local Celiac Association and she enrolled as a member, but insists that her best source of information is various web sites and a celiac discussion group on the Internet.

The general practitioner was resistant to any information that was given to her about Beryl's condition, and still is, but she did grant Beryl a referral to see a dietitian. However, the dietitian was not very informative.

Beryl resumed the gluten-free diet and within the first three days there was a significant improvement. She no longer experienced gas, bloating, diarrhea or cramps. Her brain fuzziness began to improve and there was no more need to sleep for fourteen hours.

She was hoping to get pregnant and in May, 1997 the good news was revealed; she was expecting. Her pregnancy blood work showed normal amounts of iron, calcium and potassium, however the doctor told her to take folic acid.

The next time Beryl saw her general practitioner, a request was made for an appointment with the gastroenterologist. He wanted to see her when she got pregnant, but the general practitioner said the visit was unnecessary. She does intend to remind her OB/GYN doctor of this fact when she sees him again.

Nobody else in Beryl's family has been diagnosed with celiac disease, but she recognizes familiar symptoms in some of them.

Beryl's case is unique with an odd set of symptoms which further proves that celiac has earned the name of "the great masquerader."

She has a wonderful "clean out the fridge recipe" that she would like to share with you. She says, "You can leave out any ingredient, except the curry paste, and still have a delicious dish, and if you prefer a vegetarian version, substitute the chicken with chickpeas. It is wonderful served over rice. If you prefer a sweeter curry add raisins to the rice and a tablespoon each of cinnamon and brown sugar to the curry."

CHICKEN CURRY

1 lb. chicken thighs & drumsticks (skinned)
3 large potatoes (coarsely chopped)
6 small or 4 medium tomatoes (coarsely chopped)
3 cloves garlic (sliced)
1 small yellow onion (chopped)
4 stalks celery (chopped)
2 Tablespoons Olive Oil
1 1/2 Tablespoons Patak's Madras Curry Paste
2 Tablespoons GF Beef or onion broth mix
2 Tablespoons balsamic vinegar
2 Tablespoons GF Worcestershire sauce
3 Tablespoons GF soy sauce
2 Bay leaves
1 cup water
2 handfuls dried lentils

Put oil in a large skillet on low-medium heat. Add onions, celery and garlic and sauté for 10 minutes. Watch that the garlic doesn't burn. Add chicken--it may stick, but the sauce will eventually deglaze the pan--cook for 5 minutes, turning once. Reduce to low heat and stir in curry paste, vinegar, Worcestershire sauce, soy sauce, broth mix, bay leaves and water. Add potatoes, tomatoes and lentils. Simmer covered for 1 hour, stirring every 15 minutes. If you like a thicker sauce, remove the cover for the last 15 minutes.

PAT

Pat and her family reside in a beautiful part of Southern Canada in the province of Manitoba. They have a farm in the flatlands near the Assiniboine River, where they raise wheat, oats, rye, canola, flax and sunflowers. As Pat was writing down the details of her story, her husband was outside combining rye, she says, "How's that for living on the edge?" Also, they raise beef cattle and her husband operates a small farm machinery repair service with no time for boredom in Pat's household.

Pat's heritage is a little bit of everything, including Anglo-Saxon, Irish, Scottish, English and Welsh. This mixture certainly makes it easy to figure out that celiac may be lurking in her past somewhere, waiting to emerge again. In the following story, you will see just how the disorder surfaced in Pat's generation.

As a child Pat remembers being thin, short and very whiny. She thought no body liked her and felt that she didn't "belong." She always had the feeling that something was wrong with her stomach. Her mother was a registered nurse who believed that you only went to the doctor when you were in dire straits. Thus, her malady went unchecked for years.

As a teen she was very late in maturing and still felt like somewhat of an outsider, not belonging. At about 17 years of age she started to feel better and her symptoms were easing up. She seemed to "grow out of it." At the age of 18 she decided to donate blood, but she was turned down because of being anemic which started a long history of iron supplements. She didn't worry too much about this because this seemed to be a family trait; her mom's blood was chronically low, as well as her older sister's.

Pat was to going to get married, but just before the ceremony she had some barium x-rays done to try to figure why she had heartburn, gas, etc. The tests results turned up nothing of any significance and no firm diagnosis was given.

She then proceeded to get married and had two healthy pregnancies, but the third one was not quite so healthy. She lost weight in her arms and legs, gaining only 16 pounds throughout her entire pregnancy, but delivered a beautiful eight and one half pound baby boy. By the time everything was calculated, the bottom line was that Pat had actually lost weight and she could not seem to gain it back. Still, she was anemic and began to have diarrhea more and more. Making trip after trip to the doctor to have her blood tested, she could get no answers. The only theory the doctor could arrive at was that all her symptoms were due to stress. Deciding her blood levels were normal for her, the doctor told her they were where they were meant to be. So, for ten years, or more, Pat struggled, functioning under the illusion that stress was making her sick all the time. But, in the back of her mind she was convinced that she must have cancer, and by the time it would detected it would be too late; the thought was overwhelming.

In March of 1993, Pat's sister had her fourth child. The sister, like Pat, had lost weight during the pregnancy to nourish the baby; persistent diarrhea developed and no medication would control it. She decided to find a new general practitioner, since the family's old one had recently retired. The new GP finally referred Pat's sister to a gastroenterologist. About the same time, Pat ran out of folic acid and iron sulfate and decided to make an appointment with the same new GP, who ordered some blood tests for her. The test results indicated Pat's hemoglobin levels were lower than usual. The GP was concerned. Meanwhile, at the same time, he was also trying to figure out what was causing problems for Pat's sister.

It was like a puzzle falling into place when the general practitioner realized that he was treating sisters who for years had the exact same symptoms, diarrhea and anemia, which started at the same age for each of them (age 31). The general practitioner then referred Pat to the same gastroenterologist that her sister was seeing. And, the rest was history. Pat says, "In fact, I guess it all is, Right?"

The gastroenterologist then scheduled tests for both sisters about the same time. Pat had her biopsy on September 23, 1993 and both tests came back with the same results: celiac disease. "It was like being born again," Pat states.

The GP was not familiar with the gluten-free diet, so he gave both Pat and her sister a referral to a dietitian, who was a great help. The dietitian predicted that both of them would know more about the celiac diet in the next few months than she would ever know. The GP did not prescribe any more supplements, but Pat continued the folic acid and iron for a few more months.

Within a short time of starting the gluten-free diet, Pat started feeling great. In the small town where they lived everybody had heard the news of the sister's diagnosis. Pat learned of a neighbor who almost died before being diagnosed with celiac disease about ten years before. She contacted the neighbor who referred Pat and her sister to the local celiac support group located in a nearby town; they both enrolled.

Since going on the gluten-free diet Pat has gained weight, "Too much," she remarks. She feels much better and now has muscles where she didn't even know there were supposed to be muscles. Her husband says, "I feel like I got a new woman." Pat's whole family is very supportive and, except when eating out, she has no complaints. She has to plan ahead for her at home meals as the nearest source of gluten-free flours is about 75 to 80 miles away.

Getting information about celiac to the general public is a big priority for Pat. She says "The public needs to be educated so they can understand this is not a fad diet that celiacs are on and that we cannot cheat, even a little; unlike other diets."

Pat recommends several books that have helped her very much, one is <u>Celiac Disease-Need a Diet For Life</u>, published by the Canadian Celiac Association. The other, which she relies on the most, is a cookbook <u>Gluten Free Anytime</u>, by Joyce Friesen and Donna Weld.

Pat has a delicious recipe for corn muffins that she is willing to share with you--and it's easy.

CORNMEAL MUFFINS

Sift together:
7/8 cup white rice flour
1/4 cup cornmeal
1/4 cup white sugar
4 teaspoons gluten-free baking powder
3/4 teaspoon salt
2 eggs
1/4 cup oil

In a separate bowl, beat the eggs(remove 1 yolk) and the oil. Add dry ingredients and beat together. Immediately pour into greased muffin tins and bake approximately 10 minutes. Makes 10 to 12 muffins.

CAROLYN

Carolyn is descended from Irish and German heritage. She resides in Iowa, near Iowa City, where the local university has an excellent medical clinic which is completely accessible to everyone.

It seemed to Carolyn that she was pretty healthy all of her life until she started to think back about her childhood. She was always very thin, and recalls at the age of four she fell and could not get up or walk. This incident stuck in her mind for many years. Her mother took her to several doctors in a large city. One incident with a doctor in the city was quite traumatic as she says, "He yelled at me and said that I was putting it on." Carolyn remained in the city with relatives, and a chiropractor came to the house every day to check on her. Carolyn states, "Strange, but I don't remember the day that I could walk again."

Carolyn questioned her parents about the ordeal after looking at some family pictures; she looked like a poster child from a third world country in them. Her mother's only answer was, "The doctor told me that you were "malnutritioned" and the "chiro" worked on your liver!" All this happened around 1945.

Carolyn is sure that her mother was embarrassed that her child had become malnourished and after reading more about celiac Carolyn says, "I'm sure that it wasn't her fault."

Carolyn has a theory of why her celiac was triggered; she had two very stressful years between 1995 and 1997. She explained that she and her husband built a house, which is stressful under the best of circumstances, but then each of her three children moved. One of the children moved not just once, but three times. They helped each time. Carolyn says, "These were not just across the street moves, but from

Kansas City to Minneapolis; Kansas City to Iowa, to Chicago, etc."

During that time one of the children got married and had a child. And, to add to her already hectic life she and her husband moved from their two-story home of twenty-nine years. It had to be cleared out and all the possessions that the family had collected all those years had to be sorted through. Much of the work on the new house was completed by Carolyn and her husband.

On top of that Carolyn says, "It was the hottest most humid weather that year in Iowa." Throughout this whole ordeal, Carolyn worked full time. She did have one "vacation" which she spent finishing woodwork and moving kids.

Throughout the year Carolyn had lost 25-30 pounds, but thought nothing of it. She said, "I wasn't surprised by that, I had good reason to." She did not gain the weight back which would have been typical for her.

In April of 1996 Carolyn's husband had a mild heart attack and was hospitalized. In June he was readmitted to have surgery to have a stint put in. This is when she started to break out with itchy patches of blisters and started having pain in her left side under her ribcage.

During the summer she had several cysts in her mouth which had to be removed surgically--not once, but twice. In November she had surgery on her breast. Cancer cells were found. Several days after the initial surgery, she was returned to the operating room for the removal of a hematoma. All this time she was ITCHING!! Doctors proclaimed that they removed all the cancer. Four out of five of them says that she does not have to have any further treatment.

Carolyn had dozens of tests with no diagnosis for the pain in left side which seemed very strange to her, knowing darn well that it hurt and there was bound to be a reason. She suffered everyday. After persisting, she was finally referred for a CAT Scan which revealed a cyst on her ovary. She says, "For a healthy person, I sure went downhill fast!"

Finally her MD sent her to the University of Iowa to dermatology; from there she was referred to the Digestive Disease Clinic where she was seen by a well known physician who is an expert on celiac disease, but she was unaware of his expertise. Carolyn had blood tests and a biopsy which both came back positive; the diagnosis was dermatitis herpetiformis and celiac disease. (Dermatitis herpetiformis is a skin disorder caused by an intolerance to gluten which manifests itself by clusters of itchy blisters on the skin. Often referred to as DH.) The doctor compared Carolyn's intestine on the scale of one to ten as an eight, ten being the worst. After some discussion, Carolyn accused the doctor of saying that she had "IT," so that he could have another number for his statistics, since he was "so into" the disease. He quickly reassured her with his kind words, and being very knowledgeable about celiac, he answered all her questions. Carolyn was in disbelief when she heard the classical symptoms of celiac, because she had none of them.

But, looking back, she recalls being anemic throughout most of her life. On one occasion, the doctor gave her a week to get her blood up or else she was headed for the hospital. She took iron pills and ate a lot of liver. Thank heaven she liked liver. She was anemic, her weight was normal in her adult life, and she suffered from several bouts of depression. Another thing that bothered her a lot was acid reflux. This went on for five to seven years; she ate antacids constantly, but gave this little thought at the time. It took her ten long years to become pregnant. Carolyn says, "I never thought twice about any of these simple symptoms until I read over the celiac symptoms list."

The doctor referred Carolyn to the clinic dietitian who gave her several handouts, a shopping list, and the name of support groups, but she insists, "I really learned the most on the Internet." She subscribed to the List, which is a group of over 2000 celiacs who share information about the disease via the Internet. She says, "I think I would have gone completely nuts, feeling alone in this thing had it not been for the List."

Carolyn has been on the gluten-free diet since April 3, 1996, and she says, "hating every minute of it." Her last antibody tested negative, but she still needs to take Dapsone for dermatitis herpetitiformis. And to top it off she NOW has diarrhea, which was not a problem before diagnosis.

Even with all her problems Carolyn says that she is thankful that she can function everyday and feels lucky compared to some people with celiac who have worse problems. She says, "Sure is a lot of things, it seems to me, happened in a short time."

No one in Carolyn's family is known to have celiac. However, she is suspicious of an aunt and uncle on her mother's side of the family who are of Irish descent and both have bowel problems. Her uncle has extreme diarrhea that controls his life; he has two daughters, one is a doctor and one is a nurse. Carolyn has mentioned to both the daughters about his being tested for celiac disease. They both have admitted that is an avenue that has not been looked into, but neither of them has moved forward to pursue the idea.

Carolyn is very dependent on Betty Hagman's cookbooks which she recommends for all celiacs. She also gets a lot of good recipes from the Internet which helps her through her daily meals. She copes well from day to day now that every thing, well almost everything, is under control.

JANE

Recently, Jane moved from America's Heartland, Kansas, to North Dakota where the winters are long with huge piles of snow which stays and stays, but the summers are wonderful; they lack the steaming humidity and heat of the Kansas plains. She loves the wide open spaces and the clarity of the air. Gluten-free foods are more accessible in this area than in Kansas which is a definite plus.

Jane remembers being very small even as a child; today she stands only 5'1" tall. She always had thin, light colored stools; not realizing that was a problem, no one seemed to worry about it. She had an allergy to several foods, including fish and sweet potatoes which was discovered by her mother when Jane was very young. She also remembers having a severe case of the hives one spring, a reaction from colored candy Easter eggs. The allergies kept advancing to the point that she had to take Sudafed every day during the summer, even sometimes in the winter; otherwise her nose ran constantly.

Jane's life seemed normal enough, except for the allergies, until the age of 34 when she had a severe loss of blood. After five long months she was finally diagnosed with a tear in her colon wall. A short time later surgery was performed to correct the problem and afterwards she weighed a mere 95 pounds.

Two years later, at the age of 36, she had a hysterectomy; then she gained some weight. By the time she had reached the age of 45 she weighed 125 pounds, a far cry from the 95 pound girl she once was. She started having stomach pains and the light colored, watery stools were still a constant problem. She went to the doctor who questioned her as to how long had she had the stools. She replied, "As long as I can remember." The doctor then concluded that this was normal, telling Jane not to worry. Several tests were then ordered for a later date, but all had negative results. No reasons were given for her symptoms. The constant pain in her stomach began to ease somewhat, but the doctor had convinced Jane, by that time, that all the pain was "in her head." Because of the move to North Dakota, she did not see this doctor again.

Continuing to feel bad, she felt fatigued and, again, her stomach pain worsened, becoming constant. She stated, "When I would go out to eat, I would vomit in the parking lot." Her dessert was an antacid which she ate like candy.

Jane convinced herself that she could not handle spaghetti or pizza; not because of the wheat, but because of the other ingredients, maybe the sausage. Little did she know that it was the other way around.

She noticed that her stomach stayed swollen and her body was covered with bruises. Even a slight touch would turn into a new bruise. She made an appointment for a yearly physical where she mentioned the bruises. The doctor ordered a blood count that indicated she was severely anemic; an iron supplement was prescribed.

Jane made it through life taking one day at a time, struggling with pain and fatigue. In the spring of 1995 she reached the age of 50; by then there was so much pain in her hands that she went for tests for carpal tunnel syndrome which showed no evidence of the disorder. Jane's father had suffered from rheumatoid arthritis for which she was tested; the results again were negative. She was perplexed; the pain remained, but she kept on going. She says, "I am from farm stock and you just keep on going."

In September 1995, Jane had an accident while getting off the back of a pickup truck which resulted in a broken right arm. This impaired her a lot; she had a hard time cooking and eating; consequently, the family had to eat a lot of fast food and frozen dinners.

40

In October, Jane and her family went on vacation where she picked up a parasite, she thought. When she returned home in November her diarrhea was constant. She tried all kinds of home remedies, but to no avail. Finally she went to the doctor who gave her a prescription for a medication, but after two weeks her diarrhea still remained. By December, Jane had lost 12 pounds (down from 132 pounds) and began to break out in a rash that itched like crazy. She returned to her doctor who ordered some tests, all of which came back negative; he gave Jane a referral to see a gastroenterologist in January 1996 and by this time she weighed a mere 106 pounds.

Even though Jane was eating regularly she could not keep anything down. She was so weak that she could hardly get out of a chair. She had to quit her job since she could no longer function; the diarrhea continued and she was still in constant pain. The gastroenterologist ordered a liver biopsy in February 1996. She had to be admitted to the hospital where a transfusion of four pints of blood had to be administered even before the biopsy could be performed. The test revealed no cancer, but it was discovered that her liver was quite enlarged. She remained in the hospital where she was pumped full of fluids which made her feel much better. When she returned home, however, she just got sicker and sicker. Within a short time her husband insisted that the doctor put Jane back in the hospital. He said, "She's dying, right before my eyes." She had lost all faculties, suffered from edema and a severe tingling in her hands, face and feet. She said, "My legs felt like they weighed a ton, and I had constant bone pain."

Jane was admitted to the hospital again in March of 1996 and an intravenous feeding tube was inserted. The doctor ordered an MRI and other tests. He finally performed a biopsy of her small intestine which revealed that she had celiac and by this time she was down to just 82 pounds.

41

When the doctor came into Jane's room after the biopsy he explained to her that she had celiac disease and mentioned, "All you have to do to get better is to eat a gluten-free diet. I am not familiar with the diet, but I have heard that it is a difficult diet to follow." Also, he admitted having very little knowledge about celiac disease. The doctor then gave Jane a referral to a dietitian who would explain all about the gluten-free diet.

Upon returning home, she had to continue with the feeding tube that had to be hooked up for 12 hours a day for three months. A home health nurse showed Jane how to maintain it. Three months later, in July 1996, Jane began to taper off the feeding tube and by the time she was completely off the tube, she had gained up to 122 pounds. Jane felt a lot better, but was still a litle weak.

Trying to adhere strictly to the gluten-free diet was difficult at first because she got confused easily and some of the foods she was eating were not gluten-free. She says, "It took me about a month to get the hang of it." She made a few mistakes which resulted in diarrhea for about seven days, then it took another three days to get back to normal. She had a good appetite, eating everything in sight that was gluten-free; by September she weighed 138 pounds.

Jane always prepared a lot of fresh food in her kitchen (except when she had the broken arm), but now she uses everything fresh: vegetables, meats and fruits. She knew very little about baking, but she soon learned.

Jane suspects that her father had celiac, even though he was not diagnosed. She feels that's what caused his death at the age of 74. During the last year of his life he lost a lot of weight and was hardly able to care for himself, often hallucinating, her mother told her. The weekend before her father went into the hospital for the last time, he went into a coma from which he never regained consciousness. Jane saw this with her own eyes. Her father's personality changed drastically when he was very sick. She would try to carry on a conversation with him and he would lose track and pause, then just start talking about something altogether different. He died in 1993. Jane was diagnosed with celiac in 1996; she will never know for sure if her father suffered from the same disorder.

Since Jane has been diagnosed, her sister has gone on a gluten-free diet which has made a big difference; she feels much better. Jane's daughter, who is 25 years old, has also gone on the gluten-free diet, having suffered from many allergies since she was a child. Jane says, "She seems to have DH, all the little bumps that itch like crazy." Jane also suffered from this symptom the last few weeks before she was diagnosed. She said, "I scratched so much that some places were practically raw."

Jane feels lucky because she has located three eating places that cook just for her if she calls ahead. She says, "It's fun to be able to eat out once in awhile." She recalls her first mistake when she ate out. She ordered French fries, making sure they were real potatoes, but she failed to ask about the oil which turned to be contaminated from frying breaded items in it. She found out this fact too late and developed diarrhea. When Jane mentioned this incident to her doctor, his only comment was, "You will just eat at home."

Jane says, "The doctor just does not understand that you cannot live your life not going anywhere, that you have to learn what you can eat and then adjust." Jane says that she has done just that, knowing that she has to stay on this diet for the rest of her life.

She has adjusted quite well and does not feel sorry for herself, because she says, "I know that I could have been sick with some disease that has no cure. The gluten-free diet has really helped."

43

Jane's husband is very supportive. She says, "My husband, bless his heart, eats my diet all the time and on a rare occasion he'll have a dessert which I cannot have." He says, "My system is gluten deficient."

Several books are very helpful to Jane and she recommends them for every celiac: <u>Against The Grain,</u> by Jax Peters Lowell and Betty Hagman's cookbooks which she says, "are a must." These books have certainly made Jane's celiac life much easier.

She is of the opinion that it is very important to find a support group, especially when you are first diagnosed because this is the time you really need help and support to lead a gluten-free life. She says, "It is good to get together with other celiacs, just so you can remember that you <u>are</u> normal. And, best of all, are the picnics where you can enjoy a plate of warm gluten-free food."

Jane also stresses that it is a lot easier to follow a diet if your life depends on it. She says, "I know I would never cheat, for I know just how sick I can get and nothing is worth that feeling."

One of Jane's favorite gluten-free dishes is always shared with her fellow celiacs and their families at the picnics; she would like to share this recipe with you. The recipe is delicious and it's good for you!!

JANE'S SPINACH AND RICE DISH

1 cup rice steamed for 45 minutes in
1 cup chicken broth and
1 cup water. You can steam the rice in 2 cups of water, if
you wish.

Then sauté:
1 Tablespoon butter
1 chopped onion
1 clove chopped garlic
8 ounces sliced mushrooms

To this add:
2 boxes frozen spinach (thawed)
1 to 2 Tablespoons lemon juice

Mix well and reduce any liquid by cooking. Serve as a side
dish.
Salt and pepper to taste.

PAUL

Paul lives in the beautiful country of England, not too far from London. The incidence of celiac disease is quite high in this area of the world where an accurate diagnosis of the disease is usually not a problem. But even in England where doctors are familiar with the disease a case of celiac can be overlooked because of elusive symptoms, as in Paul's case.

Indeed, Paul had no major health problems at all. His only complaint was that he suffered from annoying cold sores every two or three months. Then there was a period in his life when he seemed to be overly tired all the time. Two years later quite by accident the reason showed up during a blood donor session; Paul was found to be anemic. His doctor prescribed an iron supplement to alleviate the problem.

After a time he had orthoscopic surgery done on his knee, not just once, but twice on the same knee. The doctor felt that the damage was caused by Paul's active involvement in sports. However, a third operation on the other knee for a torn cartilage will be performed soon, although Paul has participated in sports very little for the past two years.

Paul's brother, a doctor, who was diagnosed with celiac disease two years ago, suggested that Paul be tested. Since Paul displayed no classical symptoms, his doctor was skeptical about Paul's having celiac disease. The doctor's words to Paul were, "If you have celiac disease; I'm a Dutchman." In fact the two fellows are proper Englishmen. Paul's brother, fortunately, had independent knowledge of the disease and had access to a great deal of information which he has studied thoroughly. It was at his brother's insistence that Paul be screened with a blood test first, then a biopsy, which came back positive. This indicated that in Paul's case, he suffered from a silent, or dormant, case of celiac. disease. Paul has another brother who, after being tested, has been pronounced to be free of the disease.

Paul was referred to a dietitian, who was quite ill informed about the disease and details of the gluten-free diet that Paul needed to follow. He was floundering for information when important help about the diet came from his brother, the doctor. At last Paul was headed in the right direction. Shortly after receiving the information, Paul joined the UK Coeliacs Society which is a registered charity that produces a bi-annual newsletter and an annual booklet which lists goods with questionable gluten-free status. The organization sends this vital information to all its members.

Since Paul had no acute or classical symptoms he has noticed very little change after going on the gluten-free diet, saying, "so to be honest, I feel no different." Paul has always loved food and his lack of symptoms made it very difficult for him to follow such a restrictive diet with no apparent pay-off. It was due to this, that he recently went on a self-imposed gluten challenge, after eighteen months on the gluten-free diet, to see if he would suffer any of the horrendous side effects that he had heard about. After three cakes made of wheat flour and a Big Mac over three days, he did suffer some mild stomach cramps, a bloated stomach, and tiredness, which now makes it easier for him to follow the gluten-free diet.

Once a positive diagnosis is pronounced by the doctor, obtaining gluten-free food in England is relatively simple and inexpensive. Paul can obtain as much basic gluten-free food as he wants for seventy-eight pounds sterling a year. Included are basic biscuits, flour, sliced bread, rolls, pasta and even pizza bases which can be ordered from his excellent local chemist; the order usually takes about two days to arrive. Some of the bread that Paul orders is quite delicious and indistinguishable from wheat-containing bread.

Yorkshire pudding and pancakes are two of Paul's old favorites that he misses very much, but he also misses eating Big Macs, Quarter Pounders, KFC Chicken, and Whoppers, etc. Paul is a big pie and cake fan and his wonderful wife makes him these gluten-free treats every now and then, "When I have been a good boy, that is," he says.

East Indian food is quite popular in the area where Paul lives, making it easy to make sensible choices when eating out, because most of the dishes included on the menu are gluten-free.

Since acute symptoms are not always present, as in Paul's case, the diagnosis may be overlooked for years and years which is another case in point for more general screening for everyone at an early age. A positive diagnosis, as we all know, means the celiac has to be on a gluten-free diet for life.

Marilyn

Marilyn resides in "The Sunshine State" where the weather is usually pleasant in the winter; the summers are cooled by an ocean breeze most of the time, but on occasion the heat can be sweltering. She lives in a beautiful area that has many large, old oak trees which provide much needed shade. There are several well stocked health food stores located near Marilyn's home. She has access to wonderful medical care at a local university, which makes her fortunate in many ways, but you will see that no one has yet solved all of her health problems.

Marilyn recalls, "As a child I remember always being hungry. I ate a lot, but was very thin." Some people could not understand how such a small, wispy child could eat so much and never gain weight; she says, "I stayed hungry, no matter how much I ate. My parents were so concerned that they took me to the doctor to see if I had a tape worm." The doctor concluded that she, indeed, did not. Marilyn cannot remember if the doctor ran any tests to verify this conclusion, but she does remember having terrible stomach aches frequently, but no diarrhea; quite the opposite, she was constipated all the time.

Thirty years ago Marilyn was up to 185 pounds, "Which is about 35 more pounds than what I should have weighed," she says. Still Marilyn stayed constantly hungry. She tried dieting many times which never seemed to help, but over the years, her weight finally stabilized at 160 pounds.

About 15 years ago, Marilyn started having severe bouts of diarrhea and constipation. Then by 1993 the intermittent bouts of diarrhea had become very explosive. For the next several years she saw many doctors who ran numerous upper and lower GI tests, but the diagnosis was always the same after each test: irritable bowel syndrome and she needed to take Metamucil which never did help. In 1996 she started to lose weight, about a pound a month, no matter what she did, or did not, eat. This seemed very puzzling.

Marilyn continued to eat a lot, yet she was starving and losing more weight. She still had diarrhea, constipation, stomach and intestinal pains, excessive gas, chronic fatigue, fibromalgia and insomnia. Desperate for answers, sensing that something more was going on in her body than just irritable bowels, Marilyn decided to post a message on one of the medical sites on the Internet explaining her problem. She thought there must be a clue somewhere to help her find a solution.

After her posting, she received an answer which included information about a gluten-free diet. She read the posting carefully and, immediately, decided to try the diet.

Marilyn visited her general practitioner right away and asked him questions about the disorder, but he could give her no answers. She continued on the diet since it seemed to agree with her. She comments, "I was amazed how much better that I felt, in just 10 short days. I no longer suffered from constipation problems, no more intestinal and stomach pain. The hunger pains stopped in a few days and I had no more nausea or excessive gas. In a few weeks the chronic fatigue that I had suffered from was gone."

Fibromyalgia had plagued her for almost three years before going on the diet, but it eased up gradually, then went away after about a month. Her weight stabilized at 150 pounds.

After eleven months, on her third visit, Marilyn's doctor finally recommended that she see a specialist who was more knowledgeable about the disorder. After doing a little research she made an appointment with a gastroenterologist at a local university. The doctor told Marilyn that she would have to have a gluten challenge since she had been on the gluten-free diet so long. This consisted of eating gluten products for two weeks in order to run a biopsy of her small intestine to give her a definite diagnosis. "This challenge was simply out of the question. Wheat products burn my throat so badly and I would have to take Benydryl the whole time for it," she says. Since she has such a violent reaction to gluten, the doctor recommended that Marilyn remain on the gluten-free diet and forgo the gluten challenge.

She suffers from multiple food allergies, saying, "I cannot eat fish or any other seafood, dairy products, corn, soy, eggs, yeast, peanuts or chocolate. My diet is very limited." Trying to get some answers, she visited her allergist who said the severe food allergies were caused from the damaged intestines, but the gastroenterologist said that the food allergies were not caused from intestinal problems. Marilyn says, "Now, who do I believe?" The whole situation was getting to be more frustrating with no one having any definite answers to the issues that Marilyn faces everyday.

Marilyn's general practitioner tested her blood which came back in the normal range. She then questioned her gastroenterologist about the need to take vitamins, and he said that since her blood was in the normal range and she ate a balanced diet there was no need to take any extra vitamins. Marilyn has never taken vitamins, but she does take calcium.

Neither the general practitioner nor gastroenterologist referred Marilyn to a dietitian, so she decided to see one anyway because of her many food allergies. She hoped to get some tips about the gluten-free diet also, but the dietitian was not very familiar with celiac or gluten. Marilyn says, "The appointment was a waste of time. It so happened, I had to teach her some things!"

The gluten-free diet has helped Marilyn tremendously. Now she can really tell a difference when she ingests gluten, saying, "after being on the gluten-free diet for six months I accidentally ingested a small amount of gluten each day for four days a week for several months and it finally caught up with me and caused me some problems. I was eating the buffet meal at a local restaurant and did not realize that some of the foods were seasoned with a condiment mixture which contained gluten. I found out that the spinach and the green beans were the offenders after asking a few questions. This little bit of gluten caused my celiac symptoms to return and I started to lose weight and plummeted to 139 pounds. I was sick to my stomach and suffered from insomnia. I deleted the gluten-containing items and after about a week my symptoms disappeared again." She gained four pounds back right away.

Marilyn has access to three celiac support groups, but she says, "Since I do not drive I attend very few meetings. I do keep in touch with many celiacs via e-mail on the Internet and a chat room which I host once a week."

Marilyn's ancestors on her mother's side were mostly Irish. She remembers that her mother was nauseated very often with constipation, bloating and had constant pain in her hips and legs. The doctors could never find any cause for these painful symptoms. Marilyn's grandfather on her mother's side was thin with a pot belly and suffered from never-ending hunger as did Marilyn. She remembers that he was always starved and suffered from constipation, diarrhea and gas. Marilyn says "Neither my mother nor my grandfather was ever checked for celiac disease. In my grandfather's days, the disease was probably unknown." This leaves the question, did her family members suffer from celiac? Well, this question will never be answered. Marilyn's case proves again that a regular screening program should be implemented. Better understanding of the disorder is needed by everyone, doctors and patients alike, so that when a patient suspects that they have celiac they can be referred to the proper medical professional for confirmation.

DON

Don resides in a borough of "The Big Apple," known as Brooklyn, where many good restaurants are located. The Indian and Pakistani restaurants close by are his best choices because they offer an excellent menu consisting of tasty, ethnic food which is gluten-free.

Don was first diagnosed with celiac disease when he was 14 months old in 1951. It took only one visit to the doctor for his diagnosis because Don displayed the classic symptoms which were easily recognized. No biopsy was performed, perhaps because the connection of celiac disease to intestinal damage had not yet been discovered.

Don was put on a banana-intensive diet which was the standard treatment back then. The diarrhea eased up almost immediately, but Don remained a thin child. After being on the diet for two years the doctor informed Don's mother that her son was cured. After resuming a normal diet, Don fared well, but still did not gain a lot of weight.

As Don got older no mention was ever made of the diagnosis when he enrolled for school or camps; he does not remember much about his life that far back, but does remember this: "I did know I had something called siliac. "

Evidently Don's celiac had only gone dormant, but still he failed to thrive and describes himself as "The skinniest kid in class. I had problems running a quarter of a mile in the sixth grade." Don also had difficulty passing swim tests, but he persisted, never giving up, saying, "I had to take it slowly, on my back."

Later in life, Don suffered from constipation and smelly gas in his teen years. He describes the episodes as, "The silent, but deadly type." His teeth were a problem and have quite a few fillings. He had to wear braces until he was seventeen years old.

After high school was completed Don headed to college and he looked forward to what lay ahead. He attended the usual keg parties where beer was in abundance, and, of course, it did not agree with him. He says, "When I drank beer, I would puke." You guessed it, beer was deleted from Don's campus life.

While studying, Don discovered his old malady siliac. He says, "I stumbled on it in the dictionary and learned that it is was spelled celiac, but the dictionary just defined it as a childhood disease." He thought no more about it and carried on with his life as he had for the past twenty years, or so, eating gluten-containing foods without knowing that the celiac was still a problem, remaining on into adulthood, contrary to the facts in the dictionary.

After completing college Don made the discovery that he could now drink beer with his buddies without a problem. He commented, "I could go out and enjoy a brew now and then." However, at the age of 33 he complained to his doctor about having diarrhea after having had just a couple of beers. Since the doctor was not aware of Don's prior diagnosis of celiac disease over thirty years before, the disease did not come to mind. Don continued to suffer for the next seven years as the diarrhea became more frequent.

After doing a little research on his own about celiac disease, he says, 'I learned that celiac is a disease for life!" He then opted to go on a gluten-free diet and continued with his research of the disease which led to a list of ADD (Attention Deficit Disorder) symptoms; he says, "I see that growing up I had every single one of them! Now I know why I was socially inept." After realizing that he still suffered from celiac disease he made an appointment with his primary physician who referred him to a gastroenterologist. Don made an appointment, but it was six weeks away. Since he had been on the gluten-free diet for some time a biopsy was never made. He says, "My reaction to gluten is directly related to the amount consumed and I'd never intentionally eat it so I can be tested." The gastroenterologist agreed with Don's decision and gave him some literature about CSA/USA which he joined; he now belongs to three support organizations. He says, "Support is vital when one has the disease, and I don't see how anyone can deal with celiac with out help and support, especially when first diagnosed."

Don called a dietitian who was very unfamiliar with celiac disease and gluten, therefore he did not make an appointment. He is self taught about the diet and his research led him to a great book, Good Food, Gluten Free, by Hilda Hills.

His brother was diagnosed in infancy also, but has not resumed the gluten-free diet. Celiac disease is with you for life and this is one message that Don hopes to convey to everyone; he keeps trying to educate the public about this fact.

Don has graciously included a long list of books that may be helpful. Some are informational books; some are cookbooks. One of these books may expand your sphere of knowledge about celiac or it may open up your culinary world to new dishes. My thanks to Don for being such a big help.

BOOK LIST

Diets to Help Coeliacs & Wheat Sensitivity and Gluten Free

Cooking by Rita Greer

The Gluten-Free Gourmet: Living Well without Wheat, More

From the Gluten-Free Gourmet and

The Gluten-Free Gourmet Cooks Fast and Healthy: Wheat Free with Less Fuss and Fat by Bette Hagman

Good Food, Gluten Free and Good Food, Milk Free, Grain Free by Hilda Cherry Hills

Gluten Intolerance by Beatrice Trum Hunter

The Joy of Gluten Free Cooking by Juanita Kisslinger

Against the Grain by Jax Peters Lowell

The Wheat Free Kitchen by Jacqueline Mallorca

The All Natural Allergy Cookbook/Dairy-Free, Gluten-Free by Jeanne Marie Martin

Gluten Free Gems by Noreen Moses

The Gluten-Free Diet Book by Peter and Ruth Rawcliffe

The "No-Gluten" Solution and The "No-Gluten" Solution: Children Cookbook by Pat Redjou Cassidy

The Art of Baking with Rice Flour by Muriel L. Ricter

CAN A GLUTEN-FREE DIET HELP? HOW? by Lloyd Rosenvold, M.D.

Full of Beans by Kay Spicer

The Practical Gluten-Free Cookbook by Arlene Stetzer

The Gluten-Free Cookery, The Complete Guide for Gluten-Free of Wheat-Free Diets by Peter Thompson

CAROL

Carol, who now resides in New Jersey, has been in treatment during the past several years for several maladies that she explains in her story. As the story begins, Carol recalls being told that she did not grow during her first two years. One doctor mentioned treatment with a growth hormone, if she did not start growing. Carol vomited often and was tested for food allergies, but the tests came back negative. No explanation was given for the debilitating symptoms which included rashes on her arms and behind her knees, and dizzy spells. By the time she was eight years old, every tooth in her mouth had been filled, but the main thing she remembers was the overpowering fear. Carol remembers being frightened all the time. All new situations were filled with anxiety. She says, "Only in my room, wrapped in imaginary play, could I feel some security."

She was only nine and a half years old when an incident that was very miraculous and puzzling happened. She and her family were headed to Norway by boat when the ship's engines died and could not be restarted. After a short time the ship's supplies ran low and the cook started to make bread that she recalls, "tasted so terrible that I refused to eat it." That makes perfect sense to her now. The boat drifted for three weeks, floating aimlessly in the North Atlantic Ocean. She says, "The sea was calm and the wind blew gently carrying the fresh fragrance of the clear sea air. There was no sign of land." During these three weeks Carol had no wheat products.

The crew and Carol's mom were worried because the ship was drifting with no control. Normally, Carol would have felt fear which would have paralyzed her with anxiety, but to the contrary, she felt a wonderful peace.

Carol's mother was restless, but tried to hide it. She tried to keep her daughter occupied on these long calm days and tried to coax her into some constructive activity. Her mother said, "Why don't we practice your reading?" Carol was resistant, knowing it would be another exercise in frustration. She says, "I was in the fifth grade and could not read yet." Her mother had brought one of her brother's Hardy Boys books along. Carol grudgingly opened the first page and looked at it with amazement. She read, *"Bang, bang, a shot rang down the canyon."* She would remember those words even today. Why? She says, "Because for the first time in my life I could read words without effort." All the lessons that her former teachers had tried to teach her for five years suddenly and inexplicably came together. She continued to read the whole book. She was fascinated. This sudden accomplishment, plus the fact that she mastered the Norwegian language in a few short weeks, was considered amazing by those who thought that she was "slow."

For a few short weeks the dreaded fear and the mental fog lifted from Carol's brain. She felt clear headed and peaceful. This was a short break from the anxiety that she usually experienced, but all that changed when they finally went ashore. Delicious, freshly baked bread was available which she ate with vigor. Carol says, "The mind-boggling cloud clamped down on me once again with more vengeance than before." She remembers the fears that closed in on her. Along with this she again experienced dizzy spells which made her very weak. She says, " I would begin the rituals that I would use to try to conquer the fear and try to function normally." But nothing seemed to help. Her mother sensed there was something wrong, but could not define it. Carol's mother would reach for her child, but could not help her. Carol states, "I don't think that even she understood the emotional pain that I suffered, but she was patient and supportive."

For most of her life Carol could never understand this phenomena, but now she knows the answer, celiac disease. She says, "Now, when I look into the eyes of the troubled children I now teach, I remember the pain and wonder if they, too, feel it. If they, too, are locked inside a body that is ravaged by a food intolerance such as celiac disease."

As a young girl Carol was very active, but she ate very little; then at puberty she became very heavy. At that time so very few of her peers were overweight that she could count them on her hands. At 14 years of age she weighed over 200 pounds and was 5'8" tall. She reflects, "Thank heaven they didn't give me growth hormones." Her fat was not like that of other girls who were overweight, but unevenly distributed; her skin was an unhealthy color. Carol knew she was not like the other girls and felt very alone.

As a teen Carol suffered no intestinal problems. Anxiety, depression, constant deep bone pain and muscle soreness were her constant companions. Constipation was also a problem. She suffered from another symptom: her skin would only tan on the joints, which she thought had no significance and was just a peculiarity that she had.

Carol always tried to get out of eating breakfast, but it was a family event. Her mother would always insist that Carol have at least a piece of toast and some fruit before going to school. She knew that she felt better without the food, but did not know why. After eating, she always felt groggy and wanted to go to sleep. Because of this, her family accused her of trying to get out of doing the dishes.

Each night was filled with constant nightmares; when she woke up in the morning she had the feeling of impending doom. She says, "The anxiety, which I understood had no basis in reality, gnawed at my stomach." She tried to hide her feelings by focusing on other things, but the fear and depression was always with her.

Carol coped as best she could through her teen years, and made it through. She enrolled in college where anxiety became so overwhelming that she started hallucinating, but she had a clear understanding of what was real and what appeared to be happening. The wallpaper in her room appeared to be moving and she knew this could not be happening. She said, "I knew it wasn't moving, I could feel it and knew it wasn't, but my eyes were telling me that it was. Does this constitute a visual disturbance or a mental disturbance? I don't know."

While in college all students were compelled to eat in the dining room which served a lot of casseroles, but at home she would eat mostly salads and plain meats. She said, "Perhaps that was a problem that tipped the scales, I never thought about it until this moment. But as one can see in retrospect many signs were there that seem plain now."

Carol came home because the stresses were too much to bear. Shortly after arriving home, her mother died unexpectedly and Carol did not return to college.

Soon Carol married and had her first child. She continued on as best she could, but after her second child was born, she suffered with severe pain in her legs. She said, "It was so bad that I could not sit down. I paced constantly, even eating while standing." When she would lay down her legs would constantly cramp. She was exhausted with pain. Doctors dismissed all these symptoms as psychological. Even she accepted the diagnosis because she suffered from the symptoms of anxiety and depression. Despite her inner feelings she always functioned as a responsible adult.

Since her feeling of fear was so overwhelming she was a little overprotective of her children, but she craved adventure and excitement. When she was on an adventure she says, " I could match the situation to my mood and give it validation."

When Carol's fifth child was born she suffered toxemia and eclampsia. As time passed Carol became worse. The doctors tried medication after medication which seemed to drain the salt and all the nutrients from her body. Nothing helped, and no one in the medical profession could give Carol any definite reasons for her painful and persistent symptoms.

The symptoms of her dyslexic childhood continued, but she had learned many coping methods as an adult to help concentrate. Carol re-enrolled in college where she would seek quiet places that would filter out the confusion and took extra time to do research and complete reports. She muddled through with sheer determination and persistence. Carol managed to finish college this time, graduating Magna Cum Laude.

Carol comments because children or adults may face some of the same problems, "The reason I mention my education in this article is that I want parents to see that a concentration problem can be corrected if it is a food allergy or intolerance, in this case celiac disease. This type of behavior is more common than doctors or school officials understand."

Even after graduating from college, Carol continued to have a problem with concentration. She would lose track of a conversation in midstream and could not recall familiar words which was frustrating. Carol began to have a problem with her speech; often, she would stop a conversation in the middle and not remember what she was saying. She would stammer to recall a familiar word or stare blankly in an embarrassing silence. She knew the word that she·wanted to use, but simply could not recall it. Carol remarks, "It was a strange phenomena. Before my celiac disease was discovered, people speaking to me would often begin to mirror my speech patterns." Her children were very understanding, they would finish her forgotten sentences.

Then everyone would laugh. The children would say, "After all, that was mom."

At this time in her life, one of her "things" was that she had to be in control of her environment; she had to have a car. She was compelled to come and go without restriction.

Carol made an appointment with another doctor. He examined her bruised body. Her tongue looked like it had gone through a meat grinder, her heart had an irregular beat, her muscles ached and her bones felt like they were detaching. The doctor concluded that Carol was suffering from severe symptoms of vitamin deficiency. After his thorough examination he referred her to a nutritionist. "That was the beginning of the solution to the puzzle," Carol stated. She saw the nutritionist, who her husband called "the quack doctor." This remark reflected the common opinions of most traditional medical professionals that she had visited. The nutritionist put Carol on vitamins eight times a day. She extolled with gusto, "Within one month all the fears I felt for a lifetime were completely gone. Why all of a sudden, while taking One-A-Day vitamins and eating a healthy diet, did I develop berberi, pellagra, scurvy, and other vitamin deficiencies?" No one knew the answer.

With her new found confidence, Carol did a daring thing and took a job in a high security prison where she was completely at the mercy of the correction officers. She had no fear, even though she was dependent on them to let her in and out of the heavy gates.

Carol knew that the vitamin connection was the beginning of the solution to the puzzle, although it took many more years to actually find out why. She tried a multitude of supplements and every few weeks she would come up with something else that would make her feel better. She says, "Friends and relatives thought that I was a vitamin freak." They frequently urged her to snap out of it and get a life and openly told her that she was becoming obsessive. Carol's reply was, "No one understood that when you are hanging on to your life by your fingertips, you either give up or try everything you can find an answer."

Even while taking the vitamins Carol's legs still pained her constantly, then other strange symptoms started to occur. She says, "I became extremely sensitive to environmental contamination and I began to develop food and drug intolerances."

Carol and her family moved to New Jersey. Suddenly everyone became ill with some of the family members developing heart pain and pressure between the shoulder blades. Some were breathless, but when they would go on vacation in Maine, everyone would feel much better. The doctor's explanation was that while the family was on vacation there was no stress. Carol remarked, "Little experience did he have taking eight teenagers, two large dogs and a husband, who wanted quiet, in a van, to spend a week in the woods." When Carol would return from those hectic vacations she would develop certain heart symptoms again. The family's minister happened to say, "Well it is either the air or the water, why not try bottled water?" Carol said, "Presto, it worked!" It took her several more years to discover the pressure on her heart was caused by the fluoride in the water.

Carol learned that she also had to stay away from pesticides and she began to have intolerances to certain foods that never were a problem before. She says, "I thought I was going out of my mind."

Carol continued to work despite all her health problems and quirks. The job required that she participate in a summer recreation program for emotionally disturbed teenagers. "It was over 100 degrees outside that summer," she recalls. "We walked, biked, swam, and had an arts and crafts program." Carol was on a 1000 calorie diet, and she was not losing weight, despite her five hours of exercises each day. Carol stated, "The students constantly bombarded the staff with abuse and we often were physically attacked." This put the staff under additional emotional and physical stress. Carol still experienced a problem with her speech, and her co-workers joked, "Don't sit next to Carol; you'll forget what you're saying or start stammering."

Not only was she under physical stress at work but she also went home each night, and dug four foot deep fence post holes for a stockade fence. One day Carol collapsed. The next morning she woke up and could not stop shaking. She had the feeling that she was going to pass out again or even die!

The doctor who had sent Carol to the nutritionist had moved, so she went to a new doctor. He said that she had suffered from heat stroke. When she mentioned that she had nutritional deficiencies he laughed and said, "In this day and age it is ludicrous and besides look at you." He was referring to the fact that Carol was overweight. He said, "You don't need to take vitamins, and the nutritionist is ripping you off. All it does is give you expensive urine." Carol said, "I felt degraded at his arrogance. Like so many other doctors, he refused to validate my knowledge of my body and ignored my concerns."

The symptoms persisted, and the doctor ordered a few more blood tests, which indicated that no problems existed; "psychological disorder" was given as the "old standby" diagnosis. When she asked for an excuse from outdoor duty at work because she was too weak to walk or ride bikes for several hours at a time, he grudgingly wrote, "Please excuse Carol from outdoor activities due to high anxiety." She was in emotional pain when she read the note and felt like crying. She said, "Here I was in my 50's and participating in outdoor activities all my life without complaint, and he suddenly decided that I was trying to get out of it because of psychological problems. Once again invalidating me as a human being."

The weakness continued and life was almost unbearable. There were times when just focusing on getting from one student's desk to another was a major problem. She never took any time off from work, refusing to give in to the illness. People accepted this as a sign that she was not really sick and accused her of seeking attention when she complained of illness. She says, "I worked in a fog, falling in bed early in the evening, but unable to sleep due to the pounding of my slow heartbeat." She stayed exhausted. She says, "My body had like an electrical buzz that went through it constantly." Explaining these symptoms to a doctor provided no help.

Carol discovered that salt made her feel better. (A sign of adrenal problems.) This was another piece of the puzzle that fell into place, but she didn't realize it. She went from doctor to doctor but none of them believed her story. They ordered test after test which showed no abnormalities. She still had no answers and her stomach problems persisted.

Carol felt that she was at the end of her rope, desperate for help, any help. She happened to walk into a health food store where she started talking to the nutritionist on duty who believed her story. Carol couldn't believe it; someone finally listened. Because Carol had made trip after trip to doctors who brushed off her symptoms as psychological, she was willing to try anything that was sensible to help relieve her symptoms. The nutritionist suggested that adrenal insufficiency due to food allergies was the problem and felt that she could help Carol find an answer. The nutritionist suggested an elimination diet, then a food challenge. Carol was instructed to eat meat, vegetables, spelt and soy, but she only got worse and felt discouraged. But then she tried a plan that included meat and vegetables only. Amazingly, she began to feel better, but not immediately. When wheat bread was offered as the challenge she suddenly became much worse. Another clue to the puzzle was revealed. The nutritionist determined from the challenge that it was celiac disease. After going on the gluten-free diet Carol grew stronger, but still had pain in her legs.

The owner of the health food store directed Carol to a medical doctor who was supposed to treat adrenal weakness without drugs. Reluctantly, she drove one and one half hours each way to Quakertown, Pennsylvania, where she met Dr. Posenecker.

She was very weak at that point, yet she was hyper and could not sit down. She was actually afraid that if she sat down she would not get up again. Her blood pressure was so high that the doctor was concerned. Most people·suffering from adrenal problems have just the opposite problem, low blood pressure. Carol says, "This goes to show you that everyone is unique." The doctor and his staff were sympathetic and understanding. They did not slough off Carol's dozens of symptoms to nerves or stress and wanted to get to the root of her problem. On this first visit she was trembling and says, "Because my faith was shaken I seemed unable to make the decision to initiate treatment and he had to coax me to return. I did not believe that anyone could really help me." Dr. Posenecker has treated patients with adrenal problems for over 40 years.

She had become so sensitive to everything that she could no longer take vitamins. Dr. Posenecker attributed this to from the flattened villi that thinned the intestines. He says, "This condition allows toxins to seep into the blood stream rather than being eliminated. These toxins in food cause illness and additional food intolerances can occur until the intestines regenerate." (With Dr. Posenecker's permission.)

The doctor encouraged her to just nibble on the vitamins a few times a day. She slowly built up a tolerance for them. Gradually she began eating many of the foods that she had been unable to tolerate before. Most of her symptoms disappeared, but so slowly that she cannot even remember all of them.

After two years of treatment, Carol says, "It has been a long process. I am almost completely back to normal, but I do have low days."

Every time she would feel bad she would quickly check the food ingredients, and sure enough, something had slipped by her unknowingly. This is when Carol noticed a strange thing. She said, "When I ate foods that had gluten in them, I got a sore on my tongue. It was often the first thing that I noticed; small circular patterns occurred. If the contamination continued my tongue grew red and smooth around the edges and the tongue became coated in the middle." She first noticed this when she was licking stamps, not realizing that they had a wheat-based glue.

Once she bought a hamburger patty at a fast food restaurant. Instead of giving her a new patty, the server just removed the old bun. A small crumb of bread remained on the meat. She said, "When the bread touched my tongue it stripped the textured area from my tongue." She wondered if that's what happens all the way down her digestive tract when she eats gluten. She also wondered if other people with a gluten intolerance are troubled with the same problem.

Once, someone remarked that Carol simply had a wheat allergy, but all tests for food allergies turned out negative. Each time that Carol had a bad reaction from a certain food she would find out that it had gluten in it. She says, "Sometimes discovering the culprit was a long time process, successful only after trying the food over and over; such as rice cakes." Carol knew that she could eat regular rice cakes, but not the ones flavored with caramel. The flavoring, she found out later, contained a small amount of gluten.

Carol has never had a biopsy of her small intestines and she says, "I had been off gluten for so long it could not be confirmed medically. I still get sick from one slip." She did not want to initiate a prolonged gluten challenge. She added, "I understand that many have not had it proven by biopsy. Reactions are enough to confirm the disease." Her doctor agrees with her decision to forego the gluten challenge.

Carol gradually has regained the function of a clear mind and no longer stammers or loses track of a conversation, nor does she fumble to find words. Her muscle and bone pain have diminished; her depression and anxiety have disappeared. She says, "After so many years of gluten poisoning, the adrenal weakness did not go away as easily as the gluten symptoms, and I have not completely recovered and I still cannot exercise without getting very weak the next day, but I can go about everyday activities feeling quite good. Once again many traditional doctors tell me it is just that I am out of shape. It is impossible to explain to them the difference between the normal tired and the achy feeling after hard exercise and the overwhelming weakness that comes from adrenal insufficiency. Explaining that my past record of activity speaks for itself, but again the patient's word is invalidated by most physicians." Carol still visits Dr. Posenecker regularly.

Carol believes that some of the members of her family have celiac. One of her daughters did not learn to read until the tenth grade, yet she went on to college and graduated Magna Cum Laude through sheer persistence. This was much to the surprise to all of her high school teachers and many of her elementary teachers. Her daughter is now on the gluten-free diet and is coping well.

Carol is upset because she suspects that some of her children suffer from celiac, but are in denial. They all have various intestinal problems and are overweight, but have no diarrhea. With no testing, their doctors have concluded that

70

it is impossible for the children to have the disorder and the children go along with this conclusion.

She states in closing, "I wish that the celiac disease was discovered when I was young. I hope that the next generation will have doctors that listen, research and understand the problems of gluten intolerance and other food intolerances that hide under disguises that mimic many physical and mental disorders. Perhaps it is our generation that will help this come about for those that follow."

CATHERINE

Catherine lives in the beautiful deep South on the Gulf of Mexico where seafood is plentiful. You can buy a big assortment of fresh fish, shrimp or oysters straight off the fishing boats as soon as they dock with their day's catch if you choose. The busy little town where she lives has many old mansions which are shaded by ancient oak trees, but in contrast new high-rise hotels now line the beach.

She is of Scotch-Irish descent which puts her in a high category to inherit celiac disease. Catherine has a suspicion that her mother had the disease because she suffered from stomach problems all of her life, but was never diagnosed. Like her mother, Catherine always suffered from stomach troubles and was slightly anemic. As a child she had frequent stomach aches which was so severe that several times the doctors thought she had appendicitis, but she did not.

At about twenty-five years of age she fainted a lot and felt very weak, so she went to the doctor who ordered several tests. The results showed an iron deficiency for which an iron medicine was prescribed. Ten years later she had a hysterectomy and has had several other surgeries since then, including a couple to repair a fallen bladder.

Catherine coped with anemia for many years. By 1979 she had developed chronic back pain, so she decided to make an appointment with an orthopedic doctor who performed several tests that included x-rays. A lot of arthritis in her neck and back was detected and Naprosyn was prescribed. After taking the medication for awhile she thought she was having a reaction to the drug because severe stomach pains developed and thinking it was the medicine, she discontinued taking it.

From that time on, she suffered periodically from foul smelling diarrhea, stomach cramps, and fatigue. Catherine began to have weight losses of about one and one half pounds a month periodically, which lasted for about five or six months at a time. Then as mysteriously as she would lose weight, she would fare a little better and gain it back at about the same pace as she lost it. This cycle lasted for about ten years. Between 1980 and 1989 she saw several doctors, but none of them could explain why she suffered from these symptoms of diarrhea and weight loss. One gastroenterologist performed many, many upper and lower GI tests which included a proctoscope, sigmoidoscope, and colonscopy with no definite diagnosis, just tests and more tests. She was tired of hearing the same old thing over and over, always either lactose intolerance (which she already knew about) or irritable bowel syndrome. She said, "I was convinced that they had no idea what it was." She finally stopped going to the doctors altogether for this problem.

Catherine had not seen her internist for quite awhile because she was too busy seeing the GI doctors, but she had to contact the doctor for a little emergency when she had been bitten by her cat, to ask if a tetanus shot was needed. When Catherine walked into the office the doctor realized that Catherine was very ill just by looking at her and became concerned. The doctor ordered some blood work for Catherine and later that same day, she called Catherine back telling her that more blood work was needed because the results from the prior tests did not look good. All of Catherine's values were out of range. The doctor mentioned that the people in the lab had never seen an iron content that low; her nutritional levels were almost nothing. She was literally starving, because of this condition. The internist ordered a thallium stress test and the results were positive. Catherine could possibly have a blocked artery, but the doctor wanted to solve the problem of the severe anemia before referring her to a cardiologist.

Catherine was admitted to the hospital almost immediately, where more tests were performed by a gastroenterologist. The doctor ruled out Crohn's disease. In fact, the tests showed nothing of any significance, except divirtuculitis. Since no conclusive answers were given for Catherine's condition, both the internist and the gastroenterologist agreed that Catherine needed to be referred to Tulane Medical Center in New Orleans for a further work-up.

An appointment was made with a Turkish gastroenterologist who was top notch in his field, having studied celiac disease for two years in the United States. When Catherine saw him it took only a short time to finally answer the puzzling question of her disorder. On the first day Catherine gave the doctor a detailed health history and one look at her x-rays he concluded that she had sprue. He examined her hands and the skin on her arms, questioning her if she had experienced any tingling in her hands and feet. She said yes, adding that her tongue also tingled and she had almost lost her sense of smell. The doctor said these were definitely symptoms of celiac disease which is also called sprue. A biopsy was ordered and the results conclusively indicated celiac. The doctor warned her about the inherent dangers of celiac patients being more prone to developing lymphoma, and assured her that he would keep a close watch for any symptoms that might occur.

The gastroenterologist told Catherine that she should take folic acid every day for the rest of her life. He encouraged her to eat a lot of green vegetables, especially broccoli, fresh fruits and other vegetables. She was to stay away from wheat, rye, oats and barley! The doctor suggested that calcium and a multivitamin be included as a daily regimen. Catherine was given a sheet which contained information about the CSA/USA Support Group, but very little instruction was included about the gluten-free diet. Most of her knowledge about these foods was gained from trial and error.

Later while in Houston, Texas, Catherine met a lady whose husband had celiac disease. She gave Catherine more useful information about the diet than anyone else had.

Within two weeks of going on the gluten-free diet she felt a lot better and within two months had regained a lot of the weight that she had lost. She said, "I was feeling well."

Some months later Catherine suffered from stomach pain and experienced some bleeding. She immediately returned to Tulane. After three days of testing, a colonoscopy showed that she had bleeding polyps which were removed. Tests showed that the polyps were pre-cancerous.

Some weeks later while shopping at a health food store in a near-by town, Catherine learned that another customer, Jane, also had celiac. The store owner, who was more than glad to bring the two together, relayed Catherine's name and phone number to her. Catherine soon got a phone call from Jane; the two talked and talked about their shared experiences and agreed to meet soon. Two other celiacs from the area were also invited to the get together and out of that first meeting it was agreed to start a local chapter of CSA/USA. Catherine was the first president. The group started with four members and today has grown to over twenty.

Catherine did well on the gluten-free diet, until 1994 when she developed colon cancer which metastasized to the liver in 1996. She is undergoing treatment for that now, traveling to Houston frequently, where she had the surgery. The cancer seems to be in remission so far and she says, "I feel just fine."

For years Catherine suspected that her daughter had celiac disease and recently these suspicions were confirmed with her daughter being given a positive diagnosis after an endoscopy and biopsy. It is hard to get a family member to be tested for celiac disease, especially if they do not display any outward symptoms. Going on a gluten-free diet is a hard choice to make, especially if you feel good everyday.

Catherine has a taste-tempting recipe for yummy cookie bars, which she is willing to share with us. The recipe is simple and does not require a lot of preparation time with very little to clean up afterwards--something we all like to hear, and they taste good! The parents of children with celiac disease will certainly want to try this recipe for a quick snack. The big kids will also enjoy this chocolate treat.

YUMMY COOKIE BARS

1/3 CUP MARGARINE OR BUTTER
1 1/2 CUPS OF CRUSHED POSTS COCOA PEBBLES
1 (14 OZ.) CAN CONDENSED MILK
6 OZ. SEMI SWEET CHOCOLATE MORSELS
1 CUP FLAKED COCONUT
1 CUP CHOPPED NUTS

Preheat oven to 350 degrees. In 13 x 9 inch baking pan, melt margarine in oven. Sprinkle crumbs over margarine; pour condensed milk evenly over the crumbs. Mix remaining ingredients and sprinkle them over condensed milk, pressing them down firmly. Bake about 30 minutes or until lightly brown. Cool. Cut into bars.

RON

Ron hails from Canada and even though he lives in the far north, he enjoys a warm climate compared to other parts of the country, especially the more northerly areas of Western Canada. The Rocky Mountains are nearby and warm Chinook winds from the Pacific Coast blow sporadically throughout the winter which makes the winters rather pleasant. In the winter, summer, and fall the grass is usually brown, but when covered by snow in the winter it is altogether different. The drab environment becomes a peaceful haven which casts a sense of serenity out to the inhabitants to enjoy. The wind is a constant companion to the landscape, sometimes carving out strange sculptures in the snow which makes the scenery interesting and ever changing. Ron loves where he lives, but he says, "In the future I hope to reside in an area where the weather is less harsh."

Ron's ancestry is an interesting blend: Irish, Scottish, Welsh, French, Native American and German. He says, "Perhaps more, I don't know."

Ron's health has been a problem all of his life. His problems started at a very young age and followed him throughout his life, progressively getting worse as the years passed. Before his first birthday, Ron suffered a severe case of pneumonia and was hospitalized. He was, otherwise, a very quiet baby, but has always been a very picky eater, refusing many foods at a very early age. It seemed that his brain was signaling to his body that certain foods were not meant to be eaten by him. Strange, even as infants, we sometimes can sense these things. As school age approached, Ron's health did not improve. He was sick quite often and missed a lot of school.

His behavior was a problem both at home and at school. Many people labeled Ron as just a spoiled brat. Little did they know that celiac was the culprit and no matter how hard Ron tried to conform, something had a greater hold on his body, making it rebel at every turn. Ron still refused certain foods and was even ungrateful at times for special treats that were baked for him, like pies and cakes. He opted to choose rice pudding over the foods that contained gluten; without realizing it, his brain was again signaling his body not to eat what his body could not tolerate.

When Ron was in the seventh grade he was offered some wheat kernels which he chewed up and swallowed. Shortly afterward he vomited in class. He was taken to the doctor and the diagnosis was "colicky appendix." The vomiting would become a ritual for him almost every morning throughout his teen life. He was taken to the doctor several times but the diagnosis was always the same, nervous stomach. During his teens Ron developed a problem going to sleep, then sleeping fitfully when he did doze off. The lack of sleep created another problem; he was hard to wake up in the morning. Since getting up in the morning for school was such a challenge, Ron felt wrung out like a wet towel with the queasiness and vomiting still persisting. He said, "I was always cranky." He was taken to the doctor and the diagnosis this time was that he was emotionally disturbed. This was a burden, especially for a teenager.

As Ron got older, his health steadily deteriorated. Along with vomiting every morning he began to have uncontrollable fits of coughing, tremors, dizziness and grogginess. All these symptoms only fueled his crankiness. It was hard for him to get along with anyone. His doctor gave no explanation for his symptoms, only declaring that the boy's emotional state was worsening.

To only add to his misery, he developed an ulcer, which was not detected by an x-ray. The advice from for the doctor was always the same; it was stressed over and over to Ron to work on his self-discipline, so that he could overcome his emotional flare-ups.

After a tumultuous teen life, Ron finally dropped out of high school and left home. Now he could make his own food choices everyday without dealing with the stress of facing meals that had food his body rejected because it could not tolerate them. With this modification of diet and less stress, many of Ron's health problems seemed to resolve themselves, but he was criticized often for his odd dietary choices. His doctors and family still insisted that he needed to work on his "self discipline." Ron had also taken up smoking cigarettes, which seemed to make him feel better.

For the next twenty years Ron's life seemed to roll by without any major problems. Ron said, " My health waxed and waned." Finally in 1993 Ron's general practitioner recommended that he see a gastroenterologist who, after hearing Ron's medical history ordered several tests which included a biopsy of the small intestine. The results of the biopsy revealed that Ron had celiac disease. After many years of being labeled as emotionally disturbed, this diagnosis was quite a relief. The specialist was quite knowledgeable about diagnosing the disorder and recommended that Ron contact the Canadian Celiac Association, which he joined.

After about two months Ron saw a dietitian, but he had already obtained information about the gluten-free diet through the Celiac Association. Ron says, "The gluten-free diet has helped immensely." No longer is he forever prompted to be on his toes about his self-discipline; he seems like a different person emotionally and physically.

Since Ron has been positively diagnosed, several other family members have been diagnosed including his mother and daughter. At least his daughter will not have to suffer in silence with bouts of mis-labeled maladies as did Ron; she has a headstart to a healthy life. Ron says, "My brother and father probably had it, too. Dad bled to death intestinally, and my brother died of lymphoma after testing positive for AGA antibodies."(Positive AGA antibodies is an indication of celiac disease.)

Ron returned to school and continued on to college. He is very active in the Canadian Celiac Association and has written numerous papers that have been published about the disease. His hopes are that in the near future a general screening, at an early age, will be implemented in Canada, so that no other child has to suffer throughout childhood as he did. Ron has two books that he thinks that you may enjoy: Cooke & Holmes, Coeliac Disease; and Lloyd Rosenvold, Can A Gluten-Free Diet Help? If So How?

His story certainly illustrates the problems that youngsters face when they go through life undiagnosed and demonstrates the need for early testing. This is a goal that we all must try to attain in Canada and the United States.

BOB

Bob resides in Baltimore where seafood is plentiful and many gluten-free choices can easily be made by a celiac in local restaurants without worry. Baltimore is just a stone's throw from the nation's Capitol and many residents commute to Washington, preferring the more casual lifestyle that is offered in the Maryland area. The local aquarium, where the exhibits are diversified, is popular with locals as well as tourists. The beautiful Maryland shore lures many people each year where young and old enjoy all the entraining and educational attractions.

Bob doesn't remember exactly when he was diagnosed with celiac the first time. He relates, "I have been told it was at an early age, perhaps when I was five or six years old." Then a number of years later, the doctors informed Bob's family that he had outgrown the disorder. Gluten-containing items were reintroduced into his diet without a problem, but rather than outgrowing it, the disease had probably gone into a dormant stage.

Bob's health was quite stable, until he reached the age of 26 or 27 when he suffered from a collapsed lung. He recovered from this episode rather easily with no lasting side effects. His health remained stable with no major problems for the next twenty years or so. Then he started having intermittent bouts of diarrhea, but they could be controlled with Immodium. These episodes would come and go for a number of years, but finally they escalated to uncontrollable diarrhea that would not wane.

In 1995 he decided to make an appointment with his internist who, after reading the medical history, recommended that Bob see a gastroenterologist. An appointment was made promptly and several tests were ordered. After the tests were performed, Bob commented,

"The specialist did a colonscope and the typical crap, but no biopsy of the small intestine was done." The specialist, after getting the results of the tests, said to Bob, "Good news, you don't have cancer, but we don't know what's causing your problem." The doctor then suggested that Bob have a total blood work-up and he ordered a CAT Scan. The doctor added, "You're not sick."

Before Bob would agree to these tests, he asked the specialist to look up the word celiac in the medical dictionary and the doctor gladly agreed. After a short time had passed, Bob got a phone call, "Congratulations, you have celiac," the doctor announced sounding like a best friend praising Bob for some special achievement. Bob said, "What, now?" The doctor's reply was, "Don't eat bread."

Neither the internist nor the gastroenterologist seemed to be knowledgeable about celiac and they made no further recommendations at that time. Bob was floating in a world of gluten looking for a helping hand to rescue him, but the help was no where to be found. The situation was overwhelming, but Bob was not going to drown in a sea of pity or gluten, so he started investigating on his own. He called the headquarters of many major food chains asking about obtaining gluten-free food, but no one seemed to know anything about gluten and they seemed not to care. Bob had absolutely no support locally or nationally. In his panic he called the FDA, food manufacturers, and suppliers where he eventually ran into someone who was familiar with gluten. They gave Bob a positive response which included some information about the Canadian Celiac Association. After getting in touch with the group they responded in a timely manner with the much needed support which consisted of food lists and their handbook which was very comprehensive, including recipes and other vital information. Bob said, "I had to re-invent the wheel for the first four or six weeks after receiving the information."

Bob made a trip to Canada where he had arranged to meet the Executive Officer of the Canadian Celiac Association. Their meeting lasted over four hours and all of Bob's questions were answered in detail by the Canadian contact. Since Bob had such a difficult time locating some one who would answer his questions he suggests that training should be done on the local level in the U.S., so newly diagnosed celiacs will have information readily available.

Bob then located a local support group and he is now very involved. One of his objectives is to educate the public about celiac, but he is more into the education of the lifestyle of people with celiac rather than the medical or technical aspect. Finding new sources for products and educating chefs in restaurants is his top priority. Many workers in local restaurants are more knowledgeable about the dangers of gluten to a celiac, thanks to Bob. Now many chefs in the Baltimore area will pan fry seafood separately to accommodate customers with celiac. His latest quest is to try to locate a restaurant in his area which will make a gluten-free pizza for over the counter sales.

A favorite of Bob is the crab cakes which are famous in this area of the country. He also enjoys the boiled seafood that is in abundance, usually a safe choice for a celiac who chooses to eat out.

Bob plans a gluten-free getaway each year in the Bahamas for celiacs from all over the country. This group, many of whom have never met when they arrive, immediately bond to form new friendships. These vacations always provide a relaxing and enjoyable atmosphere because the group can eat together, not having to worry about the contents of the food. The chef usually prepares special gluten-free desserts for the group and, of course, a gluten-free pizza party is always included.

Bob has a favorite rice cracker that he located while on another trip to Canada. He says, "This particular rice cracker comes from Hong Kong. They were so delicious that I wanted to order some direct, but no dice. It took a year of tenacious wheel squeaking to get the crackers sold to me directly." Bob's wife contends that they are a staple for him.

"My heritage is Lithuanian, German, and Austrian. Basically European, and to my knowledge no one else in my family has celiac," he says.

The gluten-free diet has made a tremendous difference in Bob's life and has certainly opened the way for a lot of new friendships. These new friends appreciate the effort that Bob goes through to plan gluten-free events. He recommends all of Betty Hagman's cookbooks and Jax Peter's <u>Against the Grain</u> for reading.

BARRIE

Of English descent, Barrie's great-great grandparents migrated to New Zealand over a hundred years ago. His great-grand father set up business in 1874 as a grain merchant, making his livelihood from selling gluten-containing grains! The business continued until 1973. Barrie resides in a beautiful area of Christchurch, New Zealand, in the South Island which is described as a Garden City. The beautiful flora and tranquil atmosphere attracts tourists from all over the world. When it is winter in the Northern Hemisphere it is summer in Barrie's part of the world, which makes his hometown a wonderful haven from the cold winters of the North. There are many parks and lush green gardens in the town; two rivers run through the city, the Avon and the Heathcote. Barrie lives closer to the Heathcote where he enjoys frequent walks along the riverbank.

As a baby Barrie suffered from colic quite a bit, but otherwise he was in good health until the age of about eleven. Then for over twenty years his health declined which turned around quickly when a proper diagnosis was stumbled on by a doctor who is a colleague of Barrie's at the hospital where they both work.

At the early age of eleven Barrie developed cramps in his stomach. His mother took him to the family doctor, but no reason was given for this problem. His mother was assured by the doctor that no major health problems existed, but this did not cure Barrie's cramps. He was, instead, left to cope with these painful bouts alone; he dealt with the pain as best as he could in silence.

His health steadily declined and by the age of thirteen he was lethargic, lacking the energy and zest of a normal teenager. Barrie was taken back to the doctor who discovered that he was anemic. He said, "At last, the cause of my troubles! And it was curable with iron tablets three times a day. My gut continued to grumble.........and grumble........." The iron tablets helped somewhat, because his energy level did improve, but the intestinal problems remained.

Barrie plodded through life enduring these stomach cramps as best as he could, saying, "As a young adult I eventually went off to the doctor, along with my male ego, once complaining of a pain in the gut. Not too much was said about the many trips to the little room." Again, no positive diagnosis was given; the doctor told Barrie to take antacids which were supposed to be the miracle cure this time. Barrie says, "Bottle upon bottle of aluminum hydroxide found its way through my alimentary canal, but none of it did any good. In the end, stress was to get the blame"

By the time Barrie was twenty years old he had become quite desperate. His energy was completely sapped; coping with the stomach cramps and diarrhea was getting harder and harder for him. Barrie says," I returned to the doctor, finally explaining the nature of the problem in more detail." The family doctor referred Barrie to a specialist. Barrie says, "After learning very quickly what a sigmoidoscope is used for, and what a gastroscopy involves, I finally had another diagnosis." The doctor did not perform a biopsy of his small intestine. This time the doctor's diagnosis was, "You have an irritable bowel, a spastic colon. A high fiber diet will fix you." The doctor recommended that Barrie eat plenty of whole grain bread and cereal, especially wheat bran. Barrie said, "That fixed me all right!!"

Throughout his mid twenties Barrie suffered from an ongoing cycle of intermittent diarrhea which was very explosive, then constipation, while still suffering from cramps continually. He developed another painful condition, arthritis, which began to settle in his hips. This pain only added to the stress which already existed from his trying to cope with the stomach problems. His body began to deteriorate rapidly, so he went back to the doctor once again. An anti-inflammatory medicine was prescribed for the arthritis which relieved the pain in his joints, but his stomach problems persisted.

Then in 1987, two things happened. Barrie describes one incident, saying, "I had a bad reaction to penicillin. I developed a terrible rash, swelling and was miserably sick. My irritable bowel wasn't just irritable, it was angry." Barrie's weight plummeted; he lost weight at an alarming rate, almost 20 Kg in eight weeks. (That's over 40 pounds.) He was indeed very ill. He explained the other event: "Just before the penicillin episode, I volunteered to take part in a program to establish normals for bone densitomitry in the hospital where I worked." This incident led to a big discovery; he had low bone density, saying, "I discovered I wasn't normal at all. I believe my bone density was probably always low due to a long history of mineral malabsorption."

This abnormality of his bones aroused the interest of a physician who studies osteoporosis. Barrie says, "By the time he saw me, I was a shadow of my former self." Barrie's body had deteriorated tremendously. While talking to the doctor, Barrie related his health history in great detail. The doctor quickly drew the conclusion that Barrie certainly had a problem. His immediate response to the symptoms that Barrie described was, "I think you may have a celiac problem." Barrie's response in return was, "a what???" Barrie had never heard of celiac before and was puzzled as to why his problem had not been discovered long before this. The doctor explained the condition to Barrie in detail and then gave him a referral to see a gastroenterologist. Barrie could not see a gastroenterologist right away, he says, "But I was keen to get my problem under control," so he decided to delve into information about celiac disease for himself.

After inquiring, Barrie found out even more about the disease; it was hard to believe that something as simple as a gluten free-diet could end all his problems. He says, "I immediately started on the gluten-free diet. The results after two months were astounding. The continued abdominal pain that I had lived with for so many years was gone! The cramps had stopped, and I was as regular as clockwork. I started to put on weight, and had more energy than I had had for many years."

Still Barrie found it hard to believe that such a minor adjustment in his diet would result in making such an amazing difference in his life. He felt like a new person, being reborn after almost 30 years of living in the dark shadows of pain and ill health.

Barrie never made it to the gastroenterologist. Since he was already on the gluten-free diet and had responded so well his family doctor said, "Your remarkable response to the diet is proof enough; there is no point in getting sick again for a biopsy." Because of this fact, Barrie decided not to make the appointment with a specialist and his family doctor agreed fully on this decision. A short time after getting a referral from his family doctor, Barrie had an appointment with a dietitian who explained the gluten-free diet in more detail. A calcium supplement was recommended to help replace the calcium that his bones lacked.

Recently, a bone density test was performed with positive results. Barrie says, "My bone density has improved and is now just below normal. Today my health is the best it has ever been. My tummy rumbleth no more, except when it is hungry!"

The celiac connection probably comes from his mother's side of the family, Barrie suspects, as several cousins on that side of the family have been diagnosed with various digestive disorders. Barrie says, "No others are yet confirmed as celiac, but it wouldn't surprise me at all if some are."

When Barrie was diagnosed no screening test had yet been developed; however, now there is a simple blood test that pinpoints possible celiac suspects. This test is now done in New Zealand as routine screening and is government funded. This test will help all celiacs to live a better quality of life. This cost effective solution seems simple enough, but the implementation of this test fails to be a priority in many countries. Routine screening at an early age is foremost on the agenda of many celiacs, and their doctors, in the United States; we must all work towards this goal.

On the lighter side, Barrie is enjoying life again and has a recipe that he wishes to share with you. He says, "This recipe comes from my sister-in-law and is easily made gluten-free, so long as you can get gluten-free soy sauce, chili sauce and curry powder. You can make it with more or less chicken, depending on how many people you have to feed, you can bump it up by adding more potato if you have extra mouths to feed. The recipe is easily modified by adding extra vegetables or pineapple and even works quite successfully as a vegetarian meal by leaving out the chicken."

Malaysian Chicken Curry

2 double skinless chicken breasts
1 large onion (or 2 small ones)
cooking oil
fresh garlic
GF chili sauce (or chili powder)
GF soy sauce
GF Curry powder
About 4 large potatoes
vegetables of choice
rice
400 ml tin of coconut cream (about 14 oz.)
t = teaspoon   T= tablespoon

Finely chop onion. Fry it in one Tablespoon of oil along with one teaspoon of chili sauce (or less as this can be very hot) and two large cloves of crushed garlic. Cook onion until it is just transparent.

While the above is cooking, skin and chop chicken breasts into pieces. Put three Tablespoons of gluten-free soy sauce, Two Tablespoons sugar, One teaspoon GF curry powder in a bowl and add chicken to it. Stir to coat chicken evenly. (You can prepare this in advance and use as a marinade.)

Add chicken to onion mixture and fry some more. Meanwhile, chop about four large potatoes into thick slices and add to pan. Leave the skins on if you prefer. You can stretch the meal out to feed more people by adding extra potatoes or other vegetables, such as carrots, cauliflower, or green beans.

Put enough rice in a pot to feed everyone. Remember to wash the rice in cold water to avoid it sticking. Cook rice the way you prefer.

While rice is cooking, and once the potatoes are almost cooked, add a 400 ml tin of coconut cream. (about 14 oz.)

If you wish you can use slightly less than the whole tin and stir the rest into your rice once it is cooked. You can add some more soy sauce if you wish for extra flavor.

Continue cooking until the potatoes are fully cooked but still firm. Serve with rice, stir fried or slightly steamed fresh vegetables, or with a fresh salad. Bon Appetit!!

Janet

Janet was born in Massachusetts, but moved to Texas with her family in 1969 and has resided there ever since. Janet says, "so, I have practical, Yankee roots, moderated by Southern/Texas hugs." There is a wide choice of health food stores and diversified restaurants in the area, which makes being a celiac a little easier. The support group in the area is very active which makes for a smoother transition of a new celiac into the gluten free realm.

As Janet reflects on her past she thinks also of her future by saying, "I believe my "weirdness" (celiac) has translated into finding my niche in life." Her goal is to help new celiacs in any and every way that she can. Her favorite quote, "No prescription is more valuable than knowledge,"(former Surgeon General, Dr. C. Everett Koop) sums up what Janet is helping to do for celiac.

She was born prematurely, under five pounds, in 1944. Starting very early, dietary problems were constant, no infant formula seemed to agree with her. The doctor kept changing her from one blend of formula to another trying to find a solution, but to no avail. Finally, when nothing else seemed to work, the doctor put Janet on regular milk, and she really deteriorated quickly at this point. She developed watery, foul-smelling diarrhea and lost a lot of weight. Since there was such an extreme failure to thrive, the doctor made a guess of what was wrong with the tiny infant. He concluded that the diagnosis was either cystic fibrosis or celiac disease, and went with the celiac disease. According to Janet's mother, there is no remembrance of a biopsy. Both doctor and parents were desperate at this point, as all were hoping to find a solution to Janet's severe problem.

The situation was so grim that Janet's father, who was in the Navy serving in World War II at the time, was called to come back home because the family and the doctor were not sure that Janet was going to make it. The doctor suggested that Janet go on a "banana" diet. This was the normal treatment of celiac disease at that time because the tie-in with gluten had not yet been discovered.

The diet consisted of eating nine bananas a day, along with other regular food. Janet says, "To this day, however, I am not very fond of bananas!" The diet worked, Janet soon began to gain weight, to the relief of everyone.

The doctor surmised that Janet's condition was transitory, stating she would outgrow the symptoms. Janet says, "Now, it is definitely known that you never outgrow celiac disease." When Janet was diagnosed, the medical profession did not know much about the disease.

The doctor's prediction did come true; it seemed that Janet did outgrow celiac, as her symptoms disappeared. Celiac was a forgotten word for Janet and her family in just a few short years. Her mother eased regular food into the meals and the banana diet was discontinued. Janet grew quickly, experiencing a normal, happy childhood. The only thing uncommon she says, "was that when I got a bug, it immediately went to my digestive system, and the flu stayed with me much longer than any other family member." She remembers that she was described as having a weak stomach.

The only other occurrence was that her tonsils were removed when she was a young child. No sign of celiac lingered; everyone thought that the malady had been conquered. Janet says, "I remember I grew to be one of the tallest in my sixth grade class, and felt tall at 5'7" in high school. Growth retardation can be a side effect of the malnutrition of undiagnosed celiac disease." Why some celiacs are small in stature, while other celiacs grow to more than average height is a mystery. This quirk may never be figured out. This is the celiac masquerading again, making Janet's case unique.

Enjoying her teen years, she finished high school then proceeded to college where she says, "I met my husband-to-be 'across a crowded room' at an M.I.T. mixer in 1961." He and Janet were married three years later.

Life went along smoothly with no apparent health problems, until Janet became pregnant. She says, "My first pregnancy was difficult, compounded by high blood pressure, spotting in the first trimester, and flu in the first trimester. Twins were delivered prematurely; the boy had hyaline membrane disease and lived less than 24 hours. The girl had a meningocele, was only about one pound and three ounces, but she was bright eyed. This was before anyone put the term spina bifida on these babies. She lived for three months in the hospital special care nursery with wonderful care. She died from heart failure with multiple birth defects, a blessing, but very difficult. We had genetic counseling to see if there was a reason for the multiple birth defects which included a bone disorder. No reasons were forthcoming. In later pregnancies I was monitored carefully, took folic acid and prenatal vitamins, and had two healthy children in the next eight years. Some ten years later after the last pregnancy I was rediagnosed with celiac disease. I believe now that the combination of untreated celiac disease, not completely absorbing folic acid and other nutrients, and the flu led to the birth defects in the first pregnancy. So our healthy two daughters are a very welcome gift."

Then in 1987, after her final pregnancy she began to develop bouts of diarrhea. These bouts were intermittent, she says, "It took about ten years to develop into a serious condition. The gastroenterologist did not believe I was a celiac because I was not skinny, just normal, although my blood tests showed severe anemia." Janet's doctor soon rediagnosed her with celiac disease. She commented, "The gastroenterologist was familiar with celiac disease, but I think he thought I had a form of cancer because of the severe anemia. A colonscope revealed no abnormalities, but the endoscope did show extensive celiac disease."

Janet's gastroenterologist referred her to a dietitian, but the dietitian lacked knowledge of celiac disease. She only located a few pages of information from her manual which she photocopied and passed on to Janet. Janet says, "some of which I discovered later was incorrect." The dietitian suggested that Janet go to a local library and look up information about support groups. Janet says, "She was not much help, but she pointed me in the right direction. It was my own responsibility to research the disease and diet restrictions."

Janet says, "I don't remember if the doctor talked much about my nutritional deficiencies except that he believed they would return to normal when I got on a gluten-free diet. He recommended a bone density test. At that time the instrument available was only for the ankle, but the results came back normal. His philosophy was to make a good diagnosis, refer the celiac to a dietitian and then the patient could get annual follow up with his/her own internist. My good gastroenterologist ultimately became our first Houston Chapter Medical Advisor."

Janet contacted two national support groups that she had researched at the library. The CSA/USA contacted her back first which she joined. She says, "Celiac Sprue Association USA turned my life in a new direction. I attended a CSA Conference in Cleveland in 1988, almost a year after my diagnosis. I was surprised and happy to discover two other Houston celiacs registering simultaneously, and we became fast friends. Attending all the lecture sessions about celiac disease and dietary issues opened my eyes."

Janet and her fellow Houston celiacs met with some of the leaders at the Cleveland Conference and the Texas group decided to form a local support group in Houston when they returned home. Janet says, "Since I had a computer at home,

I decided I could take care of the correspondence and mailing lists, and we could see what happened." Quite a bit did happen after this small group of six decided to meet to mail letters of introduction to area gastroenterologists. The word started to spread that support was at hand for new celiacs. Janet says, "In these years since May 1989, our members have amazingly increased to over 250. We have three medical advisors and two dietitians who assist the group. Our single meeting announcement has progressed to a chapter newsletter four or five times a year to announce our meetings."

Janet soon found out that the gluten-free diet was to solve her problems of anemia and bouts of diarrhea. She says, "It did not take long for the gluten-free diet to work although I can't remember exactly how long. I am careful with my diet and have not had many celiac bouts with diarrhea since."

The similarity that Janet shares with other celiacs is her heritage; she is of English and Scottish lineage. This is one constant that most celiacs share, heritage. We seem to be all akin in this category. Her family has no more celiacs, but some of the members do suffer from rheumatoid arthritis, which seems to be prevalent on the maternal side of her family.

Janet has worked part time since her youngest daughter was in middle school. Janet says," I only accept part time jobs, so that I can devote my extra time to celiac work. I spend a lot of hours with newly-diagnosed celiacs on the phone or taking them to a health food store, or visiting celiacs in the hospital, etc. I believe celiac disease has opened my world and expanded my possibilities. It has been good for me. I am very grateful for my blessings. I am lucky that, by the grace of God and BANANAS I did survive and thrive despite having celiac disease." Janet recommends all of Bette Hagman's Cookbooks, and says, "These are our bibles." Other books that she suggests are: Against The

Grain, by Jax Peters Lowell (Henry Holt, Publisher), Special Diet Solutions by Carol Fenster, Ph.D., and the CSA/USA Handbook and Recipe Books.

Dacey

Dacey lives in a charming little town located on the Gulf of Mexico where the beaches are white and the surrounding foliage contains many towering live oaks, magnolias, and pines which dwarf the passersby. These marvelous works of nature take on the job of providing shade which gives a cooling effect on the hot, humid summers. Gulls soar overhead as they follow the shrimp boats out of the harbor, hoping for a handout later on in the journey after the nets have scooped up a bountiful catch of tasty seafood. Many brown pelicans often sit lazily by, resting up for another fishing expedition of their own.

Dacey has not always resided in this area; as a baby she and her parents called Mexico their home. She was always quite sick and a lack of a diagnosis from the doctors in that part of the world prompted her parents to bring her back to the United States. Even after returning to the U.S., her symptoms did not abate. The doctors were at a loss as to what was causing Dacey to be so sick. One theory was that she was allergic to her formula which was changed often with no positive results. By the time she was two years old she had lost a lot of weight and had more health problems.

Gaining weight seemed to be difficult for sometime, until it was discovered that she had a toxic goiter. Surgery was performed; after the procedure, she seemed to fare better, even gaining a little weight. Dacey's parents thought that her health problems had been solved, but no one knew that celiac-sprue was lurking in her body and would surface with devastating symptoms later in life.

When she was sixteen the family returned to Mexico to visit places where they had lived and vacationed. This trip was not as much fun as the other trips to her old home because she contracted amebic dysentery and was very ill.

This was the start of the revisit of celiac after remaining dormant for many years although Dacey did not realize it.

In 1987 she went on a birding trip to Arizona and New Mexico. She says, "I began to have diarrhea which we all attributed to a change of eating habits. After returning home, however, I continued to have it, plus bloating, abdominal pain, fatigue and depression. Finally, I decided to see a gastroenterologist. Luckily, she had recently given a presentation to a medical convention about celiac and the diagnosis of celiac-sprue was made in a very short time after a biopsy."

During a follow-up visit the doctor informed Dacey that she had a calcium and albumin absorption problem, but she did not prescribe any supplements. The doctor also explained the added risks of celiacs being more prone to contract lymphoma and esophageal cancer. This was not good news and further stressed Dacey, who was already overwhelmed by the fact that she could not eat wheat, rye, oats or barley.

She says, "When I had difficulty with the list of foods to avoid and how to cook, substituting other flours for wheat flour, the doctor referred me to the dietitian at the hospital. The only real help she gave me was a list of organizations I could contact. Their informative literature helped me over that first hurdle."

Dacey began the gluten-free diet, adhering to it very rigorously. She says, " The gluten-free diet cleared up the diarrhea almost immediately, but it took the other symptoms longer to disappear."

After many years of clear sailing with none of her old symptoms, Dacey began to have problems. She discovered that she could no longer tolerate food in Chinese or Mexican restaurants. She says, "My symptoms are different somewhat from celiac-sprue. About two hours after eating, abdominal cramps and pain develop and I become extremely nauseated. This leads to a terrible vomiting spell. No one has figured out what causes this."

After many requests to her doctor, Dacey had a bone density test about two years ago. She says, "The result was a diagnosis of osteoporosis with danger of fracture." Dacey was prescribed a new bone-building drug, but the medicine did not agree with her at all, resulting in gastric pain and diarrhea. The doctor changed her medication to a spray which she can tolerate. A follow-up test has been performed; although there was no increase in bone mass, there was no further loss.

Dacey's heritage is mostly English-Irish and she comments about her ancestry, " I guess that gives me a better chance to have celiac disease. My mother was ill a good bit of the time with digestive problems and the doctors could not find out why. I guess she is the one from whom I inherited celiac sprue."

Dacey learned that celiac disease, even when dormant, still exists in the body; and the gluten-free diet must be followed throughout life. Maybe, in the future, celiacs will be screened early and educated to this fact.

DEAN

Dean now resides in Missouri, after serving many years in the Air Force at various sites around the world. This is the heart of beef country with many fine steak and barbecue restaurants available. Dean comments about one of his favorites, "They have steaks. They're high in cholesterol, by the way. They also have steak fries, they call them, but, they are really French fries. It's the only restaurant I know in Kansas City where they only use that oil for frying potatoes. So, I can eat those and not have any problems." Any gluten free food that is cooked in the same oil with breaded items should be avoided by celiacs.

Barbecue is a big favorite in Kansas City, but Dean is very particular when making his selection. Much of the barbecue is cooked with a sauce or a spice rub. Dean says, "The sauce has vinegar in it, and I have only found one barbecue sauce made with cider vinegar. It is mixed in the East, but I find it very good. I avoid barbecue unless I cook it myself, or buy it at restaurants that have assured me they cook it without sauce."

There are a lot of Mexican restaurants in Kansas City. Dean says, "The tortilla factory, where I buy my tortillas, does not put any wheat on their equipment, and I get along fine with them. I eat at some of the Mexican restaurants and get along quite good. The biggest thing that I have a problem with is the cheese. They buy a lot of their cheese already shredded, and I think they throw wheat on the cheese to keep it from sticking together. And, I don't think it is enough that they list it on the ingredients, at least they don't, anyway."

Dean relates his story: "I can look back and see that I have suffered from celiac all my life." His first recollection was when he was around six years of age. Dean was taken to the doctor and says "I can remember standing in front of him, and he was sitting in front of me with his stethoscope, and he poked me on the belly. I assume I had an enlarged belly, as is seen in the typical view of a celiac child that you find in many text books." The diagnosis was anemia, nothing else was found that he remembers, and says, "I had the thrill of taking liquid iron. In those days the way to get extra iron was to take liquid iron and I don't know of any medicine, **any medicine**, or any other thing that you can take orally that tastes worse."

As a small child he was always sickly and suffered from a lot of nose bleeds. He says, "I had, it seems like, more than my share of sicknesses." Dean had a lot of gas, especially as a child. He says, "I have even heard stories that I embarrassed my parents, as a wee one, by passing gas. That's a story that I've heard. I cannot verify this."

Even as a teen, Dean was the smallest in his class. His symptoms lasted throughout high school, but as he grew older a lot of them seemed to disappear. College days were a little easier because the symptoms had abated. He says, "After I started to go to college, I started to grow up." As he went along, more and more of his complaints waned, except the problem of having a lot of gas.

Dean graduated from college in 1950, just as the Korean War had started. He says, "I rushed over to the Air Force Recruiting Office and applied for pilot training, and passed my physical." Dean successfully finished flight school and graduated. He continued on to gunnery school and was promptly sent to Korea. He flew many successful missions after which he returned to the U.S., then he completed several tours of duty at various Air Bases around the country.

After a number of years in the Air Force, Dean began to suffer from a lack of energy. He says, "I would have periods where I just didn't feel well. I felt kinda logy. Can I say logy? Like I just didn't have any energy. And sometimes, I would have kind of dizzy spells."

He went to see the flight surgeon to get checked over. Blood tests showed no problems with everything in the normal range. The surgeon suggested, "Well, why don't you try living a little better? Like getting more sleep, do less drinking, eat a better diet, and exercise more." Dean followed the surgeon's recommendations, but still felt bad.

A base in South Carolina was the location of one of Dean's tours of duty and the beach was only about a hundred miles away. On some weekends he would drive over, or sometimes he would go just for the day. The washing of the waves on the sand and the tranquillity of the water was quite an enjoyable change of pace. He says, "I noticed one thing when I was playing in the surf, the salt water would smart the pimples in my hair. And, I thought that was really a good treatment for my itchy dandruff." When Dean returned to the base, he gave this no more thought.

After applying for a Photo Reconnaissance Training Program, he completed it by the end of 1964. Then in 1965, after becoming combat ready, he says, "I was whisked off on a temporary duty tour to South East Asia, and ended up in Thailand. It was kind of a remote base at that time, and it supposed to be a big secret. We weren't to tell anybody where we were, especially our families. Of course, I don't think they wanted the population (the people in the U.S.) to know that we were there. And, while I was there I developed a horrible case of diarrhea."

A flight surgeon had accompanied the group, and he had taken a big bottles of little red pills with him. A visit was made to the doctor who handed some of these little pills to Dean. He says, " I was to take the pills after I had flown my mission for the day and take them at four hour intervals until twelve hours before I was scheduled to fly again." Dean followed the doctor's orders. He says, "The pills sure did the job while I was taking them, but when I quit, the diarrhea started over and over again and even seemed to be more ferocious each time. Then people came up with all kinds of ideas and causes of the diarrhea, but it was accepted that travel in that part of the world was conducive to that condition. We ate at an air-conditioned airline employees club on the far side of the base." The flight surgeon thought that the indigenous vegetables that this dining hall served might be the culprit, so Dean started eating at the Air Force Mess Hall, which was not air-conditioned and very uncomfortable in the hot, muggy weather. Dean cut out all alcohol, but the diarrhea still persisted. Many of Dean's friends claimed to be suffering form diarrhea also. Dean would counter with, "How come I never see any of you guys up in the middle of the night when I'm doing the trots?"

It was hard for Dean to get a full night's sleep. He would fly fairly early in the morning and be down about noon, then he could take the pills until about 8 p.m., but when he got to bed later, the diarrhea would start up again. Dean says, "I had a couple of fairly exciting missions which might have caused extra stress. This was getting to grind on me. I was not getting a good night's sleep, and certainly wasn't getting the proper diet. I was worried about my body. I was worried about myself. And, also, we were getting shot at, so you worry about that. All in all, I began to wonder to if I had the fear of flying, and, I was getting more irritated. Finally, I thought I can't really stand this. So, I went to the Squadron Commander and told him of my situation and that I had better quit this game." Dean was returned to his home base in South Carolina where he received a medical evaluation. It was determined that he was physically fit and the diarrhea seemed to subside. The conclusion was that it had something to do with the food and water in South East Asia, and after only a few months he was assigned there again.

He served in Viet Nam and Thailand ending up at the same base where he had previously served. He had diarrhea, but it was not as severe as before. Dean successfully completed his tour of duty. He remembers his last mission saying, "When I crawled out of the airplane, I really felt weak and dizzy, boy there is something wrong with me."

Later, Dean was rotated back to the U.S. This time he went to Oregon. In 1968 Dean and his family went down to California to visit relatives where he went to see his uncle for a day. The uncle said, "Your cousin, Ron, is over in the UCLA Hospital and he is really ill." Dean and his uncle went to the hospital to visit Ron. Dean says, "He was laying in bed and I don't think I've ever seen a more pathetic sight. The guy was just skin and bones. He was being fed intravenously and had tubes all around him going into his body. Oh, it was really sad." Dean was only there for a short time.

Several months later, Dean found out that his cousin had been put on a wheat-free diet with positive results. Ron ate a lot of rice and was gaining weight. No one had any idea that Dean and Ron both suffered from the same malady, celiac disease. Dean said, "Little did I know that I was seeing a precursor of some of what was going to happen to me".

Dean was transferred back to the base in South Carolina where all the family could enjoy their weekend outings to the beach again, Dean says, "Once again I took my treatments for my itchy dandruff."

Another problem, lesions on his feet, cropped up which he thought was athlete's foot. He said, "It did itch, Oh it itched" Everyone had a remedy for Dean's itch, powders, salves and sprays, but nothing helped. The lesions got even worse. He says, "They would hurt so much that I'd have to sit down and scratch them. The best was to break one and then it hurt, and itch some more." Dean was miserable and felt horrible.

On a trip to the barber shop once, he and the barber were alone in the shop and Dean asked the barber if he knew what the pimples were on his scalp. The barber leaned down close and whispered, "It's seborrhea." It seemed like the barber was afraid to say it out loud, even though no one was around to hear. Dean tried all kinds of across the counter remedies, but none worked. He became desperate and even tried pouring salt water over his head, hoping to dry the pimples up so that he could get some relief from the itching.

Dean got out of the Air Force in 1975, but he went from one high stress job to another, the commodity's business. He says, "Sometimes, I think the commodity's business was a lot more stressful than the flying airplanes. Some of the darndest things would happen so fast and you had to make immediate decisions really fast. Afterwards you would look at it and wish you would have had some time to work on the thought process and come up with a more logical plan of action."

Dean's stomach problems escalated with the gas and diarrhea getting worse. Dean's wife, who worked as a naphrology nurse in the dialysis unit at a local hospital, urged him to see a doctor. She selected one of the doctors in the unit to be the family physician and Dean made an appointment to see him. Dean related his symptoms and health history to the doctor, who ordered some GI tests. He went in for the first test and says, "Boy, I'll tell you, I don't know about this. I knew I was sick. I knew something was wrong with me, but I was afraid of what they would find."

Dean had a cousin whose husband had suffered with intestinal problems. Dean says, "He had something wrong with his gut. So the surgeons decided they'd take his colon and reverse it so the parastolisis would go upwards instead of downwards, and they thought that maybe that would solve his problem. Well, of course, it didn't work. He ended up with a colostomy and, of course, I don't know for some reason this played on my mind." He was afraid that the doctors would try some surgical procedures on him that would not work out, so he did not go back for further tests. This made his wife worry even more. Things were not going well at all.

Dean was in agony and his feet hurt terribly. He developed cold sores that seemed to stay; one would heal and another would soon take its place. He says, "When I was in the Air Force, people would make fun of me for having so many cold sores." But now they were much worse He had medicine stashed in his desk in his office and had more at home, but none of them seemed to help. All they did was relieve the pain.

Dean tried to solve the problem himself because he did not want to take any more tests. He ran a lot and tried to eat a more healthy diet including Great Harvest whole wheat bread. He commented, "The bread was so heavy I couldn't even eat a whole slice. I put wheat germ on my Wheaties, and on my oatmeal. I ate graham crackers, because I knew they were health food. I tried a few vitamins. But none of this seemed to help and I was losing weight."

Both Dean and his wife attended a flying class reunion. He says, "Of course that was a lot of high living, a lot of beer drinking. And I **really** got sick. I was sick at both ends" This really scared his wife. He says, "She laid the law down." She told him, "You either go back and have those tests or forget about it. I don't want to hear you complain."

Finally, he went back to the doctor and agreed to go through the battery of tests that was lined up for him. He says, " Some of them were kind of interesting." Because his wife was a friend of the doctor, he would have Dean do some tests as an out patient that had always been done on in patients before. He would hang around the hospital after the tests were completed, waiting for the results. His idle time was spent reading books and talking to his wife.

Finally the doctor said, "It looks like you have a gluten induced enterophothy." The doctor then ordered one more test which was set up for several days later. Dean says, "Boy, I was really feeling miserable that day. My feet hurt so much I could hardly walk." When the doctor announced that a biopsy of the small intestine was going to be performed, Dean really exploded saying, "Good gosh Doc, you're worried about my gut and here I am, I can't hardly walk. Well, I scared him so much, he sent me over to the x-ray shop and I had some pictures taken of my feet. Then I went over and had my biopsy."

After finishing his tests he went back to work. Two days later, Dean's wife called him from her office to tell him that the results of the biopsy were back and he did have celiac/ sprue. She explained that he would have to go on a gluten-free diet. His wife added that the dietitian in the dialysis unit would give her a list of the do's and don'ts to bring home. When Dean got home, he looked at the list in anticipation. He says, "About the first thing I did was buy some rice cakes."

This was on a Thursday. Dean started the gluten-free diet right away. He says, "When I woke up Saturday morning, I don't think I have ever, ever felt better in my life. I just had a abundance of energy that I had not had for a long, long time."

Dean is grateful to his doctor. Many people were amazed that the doctor could come up with a diagnosis in such a short time after Dean decided to go and have the tests performed.

About the information that he received from the dietitian, he says, "It was not a book, it was just a slip of paper, and I think by today's standard it would be probably pretty poor. But what they knew in 1982, I think it was probably very satisfactory. Probably the best you could get."

Nearly two months after being diagnosed Dean was not doing well. He was having a rough time sorting through his problems, when one of his co-workers said, "Say, I was reading in the paper that there's a bunch of people that seem to have the same thing that you do and they are having a meeting over there in Overland Park." Dean got a copy of the paper. He found out that the local CSA chapter was holding a meeting and decided, then and there, to attend the meeting.

When the meeting started, Dean was asked to stand to be introduced. The members asked him how he was doing. Almost in tears, he answered, "I am not getting along well A-TALL." Since Dean had been an undiagnosed celiac for so long his body was quite devastated and not yet had time to heal. He had been on the gluten-free diet only a short time.

One member that was present had a note book that was chock full of the names of food items that were GF. He says, "Every meeting I was over there to study that and learn a little bit more." He also received the CSA handbook and news letter which were both helpful tools that he used to educate himself to the gluten-free facts of life.

Dean also had a CSA/USA mentor who helped him tremendously. He says, "I never did meet this mentor, but we spent many, many hours talking on the phone. He was as helpful as he could be. I would tell him how I was still having problems." The mentor answered, "Well, you know one of the problems is eating out." Then Dean decided to carry his lunch to work, which worked out well. His mentor told him he never ate out and only ate food that he prepared himself, and when he took his wife out to a restaurant, he would visit with her and drink hot water. Dean learned to enjoy hot water as a replacement for coffee and tea. Dean says, "Now, I drink coffee. I kinda think it does my gut some good, if I drink regular coffee. Forget the caffeine-free coffee and the herbal teas, because there is something in them that really bothers me."

It was hard work to maintain the gluten-free diet. Dean learned new things all the time, he says, "I guess it took about ten years before I really found out things."

Rice bran and rice polish were used to enrich his food, but he still had problems. He discussed this with Sam Wylde III of Ener-G Foods who informed Dean that not all people tolerate rice bran and rice polish well. Dean deleted these from his diet which seemed to help quite a bit. Dean says, "It took me awhile to learn about certain kinds of sugars, and toothpaste, certain types of mouthwash, and not to lick stamps. That took time for me to figure out. I read a book that was written for kids on how to find out what food was causing digestive problems. You were to start out eating rice, green beans and some kind of lamb or mutton and add one item every three days as long as the results were good. For about a week I ate green beans, white rice and lamb patties, and rice cakes. I do remember drinking 7-up because it was clear and I figured it wouldn't hurt me. Well, anyway I finally gave up on that because it was not working. Now that I go back and analyze that, I figure it was probably the sugar in the 7-up that was the problem. I do believe my gut was so badly destroyed that I couldn't digest sugar at that time. But, I kept on working on the diet and have finally gotten it down fairly decent. I give a lot of the credit to CSA/USA and I feel real indebted to those people."

Dean recommends the CSA handbook and is looking forward to the new one that is about to come out.

The gluten-free diet has helped him tremendously, even though it took years of concentration with trial and error of various foods and condiments to get it just right. Dean says, "The celiac diet certainly helps, I'm putting on weight, but my cholesterol is rising. And, I have enough energy to play tennis."

Dean went back to the doctor and asked him if all the pimples on his elbows, knees, and buttocks could be dermatitis herpetiformis. He had read about DH in the literature from CSA/USA. The doctor responded with, "I don't know," but he recommended that Dean see a dermatologist. Dean made an appointment with the referred specialist. When he arrived the doctor took one quick look at the areas and said, "Oh, yes, yes, that's DH. That's a typical case, if I ever saw one. That will be twenty-five dollars." Dean says, "I know my original doctor was expecting a biopsy."

Dean needs no medication for the dermatitis herpetiformis. He says, "I know a lot of people who claim to be on the gluten-free diet, but will still take the DH medication when they break out. I think I've gotten this thing under control now, and know I have ingested gluten when I break out. Of course, I don't know that they will ever find out what the lead time is from the time of ingestion of gluten until you have a itch some place. I just feel the medicine is just too harsh to take, so I prefer not to take it." For a long time after being diagnosed, Dean still suffered from bouts of itching caused by DH. Evidently, he was ingesting some hidden glutens. He receives many calls from fellow celiacs who suffer from DH. He says, "I have found many people who have spent years controlling their DH with medicine and now they are learning that they cannot tolerate the medicine anymore. So, they have to change medicines to something that is more extreme or go on a gluten-free diet. And, they would have been much better off if they had started the gluten-free diet years ago."

Everyone in Dean's family is very supportive of him. They all try to help him stick to the gluten-free diet. He says, "By the way, I was given a bread machine as a Christmas present by my kids, and it has just been wonderful. I use it a lot. Maybe that's one of the reasons why I'm gaining weight."

Dean's oldest daughter gave him a rice cooker. He says, "I thought, what a stupid thing to do. I wouldn't buy one of those, because anybody can dump a cup of rice into a pot with two cups of water and let it simmer for thirty minutes. There is nothing to it, just watch it a little bit. Well, after I got one as a present, and found out it is a terrific addition to the kitchen. I went to my first national CSA/USA conference at Omaha. I think it was the last one they had in Omaha, and this neat Oriental girl gave one session using rice cookers. She cooked up the nicest recipe during the session and let us all sample the results. I had the recipe at that time. I never used it and now I cannot find the recipe. I thought it was an easy way to cook a quick meal."

Dean's family is of Swedish heritage. He recalls an interesting thing that happened about his family, "about two years ago after I was diagnosed, my brother, who went to Iowa State, as I did, had a daughter who was attending Iowa. Iowa State was going to play football at Missouri. My brother and part of his family went for the weekend along with part of my family to watch the game and have a mini family reunion." After the game was over, everyone met back at the motel.

Dean gives a little background: In 1954, when he was in the Air Force, his mother had written to him describing his brother's problem with eczema. He was in real bad shape and had traveled around to many hospitals and doctors, but no one seemed to know what it was.

That night in the motel the full story was related to Dean by his brother who said, "It was finally diagnosed as dermatitis herpetiformis." This shocked Dean who said, "Roger, do your realize that condition is caused by ingesting gluten and is the same stuff that I have? He said, no he did not know that DH caused by gluten in the diet, and added

116

that the hospitals were to let him know if they ever found a treatment for it. I told him to get on a gluten-free diet, which he did. His DH improved, and his gut problems that he had for years got better." This situation proves that education of the public about celiac disease and dermatitis herpetitformis should be a priority for everyone.

Traveling used to be a problem for Dean. He says, "I love potatoes with my eggs in the morning, but I never realized what a problem this could be, until I happened to see a chef cooking my breakfast one morning. He would turn some eggs, then go turn some pancakes, then turn the potatoes, and go back to the pancakes, all with the same spatula. I learned right then and there potatoes were not for me when eating out, unless they were baked. I usually order poached eggs and grits, if they have them. I usually take rice cakes as a substitute for toast and a packet of instant grits, in case they don't have grits on the menu. I ask for a pot of hot water and mix my own grits at the table. My son who lives in Alabama, claims that instant grits aren't the real thing."

One other real touchy problem that we celiacs all face is when visiting friends or relatives and eating with them. Dean says, " When you visit people once and you come back the next time, especially relatives, they're going to fix you up and make something that is gluten-free. I had a brother-in-law who made some rice crisps and marshmallow bars. And, of course, they're made with rice crispies which have malt in them. So, now, you have this situation, and say well, I sure appreciate what you did for me and thank you for all that trouble, but, I can't eat it. It is some kind of an odd situation." All of us can sympathize with Dean because we've all been there and done that.

STEVEN

Steven resides in the picturesque state of New Mexico, just south of Albuquerque, near the beautiful Manazano Mountains. Different light seems to change the way the mountains look. It seems as though they have been freshly painted by a different artist every day; sometimes they are a soft purple then again sometimes they are brown and harsh. Needless to say, the view is a pleasure.

Steven is descended from Russian, Austrian and Polish (Jewish) roots. He has felt pretty healthy all his life, until 1984 when he contracted nonspecific hepatitis. The first time that any noticeable stomach problems occurred was in 1986, when he developed the onset of diarrhea and nausea. He thought the symptoms were due to stress or some strange backlash from the hepatitis. Thinking that eating a more bland diet would soothe his stomach, Steven opted to eat softer foods that included a lot of milkshakes which led to a weight problem. The thought of stomach ulcers had also entered his mind. Often when unexplained, aggravating symptoms persist, all kinds of sicknesses come to mind. He yearned for something to eat or drink that would make his body just feel better.

Since no specific food that Steven tried seemed to help, he finally went to his doctor who recommended a specialist. An appointment was made a with a gastroenterologist who ordered a long menu of tests to be performed which included a barium enema, lactose tests, and an endoscopy. Steven did not enjoy any of them. His biopsy was conclusive with a positive diagnosis of celiac disease. The gastroenterologist explained the basic information about the gluten-free diet and referred Steven to a dietitian. The doctor discussed the fact that Steven may have a vitamin deficiency due to malabsorption caused by celiac disease, but he made no recommendation to Steven to take supplements.

After deleting milk products and massive doses of pasta from his diet, Steven felt much better, but he occasionally indulged with a bagel or sandwich on wheat bread. The classical symptoms of celiac were never a problem when Steven was cheating on the gluten-free diet. Because he was given only a few pamphlets at the time of diagnosis and the nutritional advice was so sparce, he thought that straying from the gluten-free diet once in awhile would not be a problem. Steven's situation only underscores the need for better education about celiac disease.

Steven's liver never quite repaired itself after the bout of hepatitis, so when he went for a routine check up his doctor ordered a liver biopsy. The specialist who performed the liver biopsy explained to Steven that ingesting even a small amount of gluten over a period of time could lead to a multitude of other gastrointestinal problems. The doctor also explained that celiacs are more prone to develop cancer and advised Steven to take caution and have regular check-ups. This spurred Steven to eliminate his occasional bagel and sandwich on wheat bread. Steven then started to make a conscious effort to eliminate all gluten from his diet. He now understands that a strict adherence to the gluten-free diet for life is a must.

Steven says, "The lactose intolerance actually has been the most impressive symptom since it brings gas, diarrhea, etc., but apparently has no disastrous effects (a la cancer), and was supposed to go away once a gluten-free diet was maintained." Unfortunately, the lactose intolerance remains.

Steven was not informed about a support group when he was diagnosed, but he recently found out about a local one which he joined where he found a lot of new friends. Steven is now better informed and his future looks a lot brighter.

AILEEN

The first years of my life were spent in Alabama where my parents raised their own chickens, rabbits and vegetables. This was during the Second World War when everybody had a Victory Garden. None of the typical childhood diseases bothered me, although my sister and brother had almost all of them. I pouted when they received extra attention and special food while they were sick.

In fact, my only problem seemed to be my terrible teeth. Even though I brushed regularly they always gave me problems, especially a lot of toothaches, which meant frequent trips to the dentist that resulted in a mouthful of fillings. My dentist said, "Your decay is never ending. It runs and runs." At such a tender age, these words seemed ominous. What did this mean? And, did the decay extend into my soul, as well as my body? Terror crept into my mind when this was mentioned because the strict nuns at my school always said, "Be clean of mind, body and spirit." Was this a mortal sin? Decay that runs and runs. This worried me.

During grade school and through my teen years I remained healthy, but weakness was a problem; athletics were not my forte. Running was difficult; I would tire easily, and could not keep up with others when participating in sports. Reading was my favorite hobby.

My family moved to Mississippi when I was in the eighth grade. My life was calm during my teen years which I enjoyed. Nothing of any significance happened until my senior year in high school when I had a tumor removed from my gums twice within the span of a month. After graduation, marriage was the next logical step; after all, being a housewife and mother seemed only natural to me because back in the "fifties" women were expected to get married, settle down, and raise a family, not work. So my upcoming marriage to a young career military man suited my family just fine.

My future husband was stationed at Ft. Knox. The move to Kentucky was an adventure that I looked forward to with great anticipation, but after marriage and settling there, my life changed drastically. In a short year my first son arrived. Motherhood was especially demanding; because we lived in Kentucky there was no family support system close by and my husband worked long hours with few weekends off.

That's when everything started to go to pot. The first problem was a pain in my lower right side. The doctor explained that when I ovulated, pain would occur, but the pain was more frequent than once a month. Did l ovulate all the time? Maybe that's why getting pregnant was so easy. Who knows? As a young girl I led a very sheltered childhood and this thought came to mind.

Colds and flu began to be a constant problem. The good old days of my childhood were longed for, when sickness was never my companion. My fourth pregnancy was very hard because I had frequent colds, attacks of gas, and diarrhea that persisted. My son was born with no soft spot in the top of his head. The doctors concluded that surgery was needed to correct the problem and my prayers were that his head was just small which was a family trait. He was very active, progressed nicely, and sat up at a very early age. After two years of endless trips to the hospital and frequent tests the doctors said that he was growing normally; therefore no surgery was needed. My prayers had been answered!! Often, I have thought since being diagnosed with celiac, did this disorder affect my pregnancy? Were the problems of gastric distress because of celiac? No one will ever know.

My last pregnancy was so draining and the doctor said "you're washed out," meaning that I was very anemic. He gave me a prescription for iron tablets and birth control pills, explaining that I must get into shape because my children needed me. Physically, I was a mess and weighed only a hundred pounds or less and being 5'7' tall I was a string bean for sure!! My friends called me "Long Tall Sally," a song that had been popular.

A short time later my husband received orders to go to Vietnam, but the conflict had not really heated up yet. The children and I went to live in Mississippi near my mother who was very lonely because my daddy had just passed away at the age of fifty. He was of Irish decent and through most of his life suffered with many of the same problems that has bothered me in the past. I have often wondered if he had celiac. My mother lived to be eighty-two and was quite healthy up until the last year of her life. She was of French and Indian descent.

Shortly after arriving in Mississippi, I began to have uncontrollable diarrhea which lasted for almost a week. The doctor said that hospitalization was the only answer because I was dehydrated. Tests were made, but nothing conclusive was decided. The doctor finally came up with a theory that he called "Vietnam Wife Syndrome." He explained that sometimes when a husband left suddenly, in many cases, the added stress would set off intestinal problems. Looking back, was this a bout of celiac disease? No one will ever know.

My doctor recommended that I look for a job to occupy my time; he mentioned that if I could not find one he would put me to work in his office, but within a week I obtained a position at a local department store. Then I hired a wonderful lady to come to my house everyday to take care of the children, clean and cook. This arrangement worked very well. Every week when I cashed my payroll check most of it was paid to the baby-sitter because my work was considered therapy and it was certainly cheaper than a shrink. Severe colds seemed to plague me, but taking a day off work was not my nature.

After about two years my husband returned from his overseas assignment. We moved to Georgia and for years my life rolled right along with relatively few problems, except frequent colds and flu. Then one morning about five a.m. I woke up with stomach pain and vomiting. I made a trip to the emergency room thinking the flu had struck again, but the diagnosis was a surprise to me. Blood tests revealed that my white blood count was high and combined with my other symptoms the doctor concluded that I had appendicitis. Surgery was done later that day. After the operation, when I was coherent enough to talk, the doctor stopped by my room with some enlightening news; he explained that my appendix was not inflamed, but it was removed anyway and it was located on the wrong side which resulted in an incision all the way across my abdomen rather than the usual two inch one. Looking back, were these unusual events caused by celiac? Again, this question goes unanswered.

In my research, several other celiacs have stated their white blood count has gone up at different times in their lives for no apparent reason, but they did not have surgery because the high white count was not accompanied with any other symptoms

Some time later, I had a hysterectomy after years of suffering from excessive bleeding and cramps. The doctors said that thirty-five was too young for a female to have that surgery, but because several pap smears had bad results the operation was performed anyway. I was so weak and anemic by the time of surgery that I had to be transported by wheelchair from my house to the car, and then into the hospital, because walking, even a short distance, was impossible.

It seemed that anemia was a constant problem and blood tests were performed often. On several occasions after the needle was withdrawn from my arm, blood spewed from the tiny puncture like an oil gusher, but no one seemed concerned. Were these experiences brought on by a lack of vitamin K because of malabsorption as a result of celiac disease? We'll never know.

Colds and the flu still seemed to be a problem and, for no apparent reason, I had short bouts of intermittent diarrhea which brought on extreme fatigue. Headaches started to plague me every day and I had a constant temperature of about one hundred degrees that persisted. My energy was sapped; even walking was a major task. After several months and numerous tests, a panel of doctors at the military hospital came to the conclusion that all I needed was complete rest for at least six months. These symptoms were attributed to stress which seemed plausible.

Thank heavens for my brother who said that I could come and stay with him for as long as I needed to recuperate. He had a live-in housekeeper who allowed me to unwind and get the rest that I needed. His house was a wonderful stress-free alternative, where I was able to relax without any worry. The peace and tranquility helped to ease my stress and heal my body.

My husband, who had retired from the military, and children went to Florida to stay with grandparents for the summer. The children were teenagers and two of them had completed high school. The older boys opted to stay in Florida to work and attend college where they remain today. The other two boys returned to high school in Alabama, where their dad had obtained a job. Since my six months rest was not complete I remained in Mississippi and I made a decision to file for divorce.

About a year rolled by and wellness had become a welcome part of my life. That's when George, my present husband, entered the picture. This was like a breath of fresh air for me after years of illness and uncertainty which seemed to have a stifling affect. We talked on the phone a lot since he lived about 200 miles away. He came to see me on the weekends and in one conversation I mentioned that a traveling saleslady's job would be a perfect way for me to see him more often, then he commented, "Why don't you just travel down here and stay full time?" This was a round about way to propose. We were married a short time later, and I moved to the Mississippi Coast where we reside today.

A few months later, George suggested that going back to college might be an interesting change of pace for me, so I enrolled in a local college soon afterwards. This experience was thoroughly enjoyable until I began to have severe back pain that radiated down my left leg. Nothing seemed to help. Pills only dulled my senses making it hard to study. Graduation was my goal, "come hell or high water," and after many long months, it soon arrived.

A great job at a local chemical plant opened up; I decided to take it, but after working there for about a year my voice got real raspy. On Monday morning talking was not a problem, but by Friday afternoon my voice was hardly audible and my throat felt like sandpaper. Then other items became irritants which included ink from the newspaper, leather, perfumes, etc. I thought that chemicals at the plant had set off this sequence of events so I resigned. Would this never end? Mystical maladies seemed to be a scourge in my life, just ebbing now and then giving me a false sense of hope that my life might be normal. Each tidal wave of sickness seemed to loom larger than the one before.

After visiting several allergists with no positive results, I made a trip to a clinic in Mobile where the doctor diagnosed me with candida. The treatment was a self-administered shot every day, but relief lasted only for about an hour. Not knowing how these shots would affect my body in the long term, I discontinued them and the allergies persisted. The doctor then ordered a panel of food allergy tests which indicated that a wheat allergy existed. Wheat products were cut out of my diet I thought, but unwittingly, gravies and breaded items were still included.

I visited allergist after allergist with no solution to the problem. One doctor diagnosed me with chronic fatigue syndrome and recommended that I take it easy. Another thought possibly that asbestosis was the problem, but an x-ray proved negative. Still later, another doctor did an exploratory procedure of my throat and lungs. He found nothing of any significance, but the allergies were still there. Suffering seemed to be unending. It was hard to go out in public places because even slight odors bothered me.

As time went on, the tidal wave of ill health swept over me once more. Because I had uncontrollable diarrhea, the doctor ordered tests which revealed a parasite. After about a month, and two rounds of medication, further tests indicated that the parasite had cleared, but my weakness and fatigue remained.

Driving home one evening, while I was sitting at a red light, a huge, older model vehicle rammed into my car. All I can remember about the wreck was a big boom and being hauled off in an ambulance. Tests were made at the hospital which indicated that no major harm had been done and after a couple of hours I was released. A problem did remain; apparently the force of the accident jolted something in my back, because I cannot sit for any length of time. This has been a problem for me ever since then.

Several months went by before the tidal wave of diarrhea swept back into my life again. The doctor thought that I had parasites again, but tests were made and the results were negative. Dehydration was the main problem, so I was hospitalized with drips for several days and no specific diagnosis was given.

The pain in my back worsened, so my internist recommended that I see an orthopedic doctor who ordered an MRI. The test was performed about a week later; a herniated disc in my spine was revealed which resulted in my being hospitalized for about month on bed rest which did not help at all. Surgery was the only alternative, but anemia was a problem. The operation could not be performed until my blood count increased, so I was sent home with a prescription for iron pills. After about ten days the surgery was performed; my strength was sapped and my recuperation was long and arduous. My muscles had melted away during my idleness in the hospital, which made walking a chore.

I related the story about my allergies to a friend. She told me that her granddaughter had a similar situation and the doctor instructed her grandaughter to eat yogurt with active cultures, so I tried it. This was a godsend because my allergies subsided somewhat. Reading the paper was no longer a problem, although some perfumes and cigarette smoke still bothers me.

The back surgery helped somewhat, but I still suffer from constant lower back pain to this day. After several years the pain worsened and my bones and joints began to ache tremendously. Frequently, my whole body felt like it was hooked up to an electrical outlet because every nerve ending would surge with a burning pain. This seemed like I had a million, minute burning sparks under my skin.

Later, my neck began to bother me and an MRI revealed a bone spur which was inoperable. Then my knees started to give me trouble. The doctor ordered physical therapy, but it seemed to be a waste of time, as nothing helped. By then my left leg started to drag like it was partially paralyzed, but no one seemed to know why. Finally, I saw a new doctor who specialized in knee problems and he made a diagnosis of softening of the cartilage around my knees. He also explained that the muscles in my legs were very weak which caused the knee bones sit out of place, rubbing bone on bone. Because of the pain, sleep was impossible.

This doctor ordered more physical therapy, but it did not seem to help. I returned to my internist for advice and he said, "Aileen, if I could, I would get you a skeleton transplant." These words I will always remember and appreciate for the rest of my life. The care and sympathy that he gave me, even though he could not solve my never-ending problem with pain, will always be a positive memory. His compassion and kind words helped when no medication would. Drugs just made me dizzy and drunk, but the pain remained. Opting to bear the pain, I deleted the drugs.

Since my health was deteriorating, I decided to retire from the work force permanently. Day to day problems seemed harder and harder to cope with because of the pain and for that reason retirement seemed to be the only answer.

About a year after retiring I started to gain weight, ballooning up to 150 pounds according to my bathroom scales. A slight swelling with tingling in my extremities became a problem, and my rings were hard to remove. My hair had become so dry and unmanageable that it looked like dead grass that had been cut with a weedeater. Also, my skin was very dry and it resembled the skin of a sun-baked crocodile. Every time something touched my body a bruise would appear; it looked as though hundreds of purple polka dots were painted on my skin. At night, sleep was elusive. And if it came, often times it would be interrupted by a strange occurrence; when I awoke in the middle of the night my hands would be absolutely numb which was frightening.

One morning on my way to the bathroom my head reeled which made walking impossible. It was a good thing that the wall was close; just hanging on to it was quite a task. Thank Heaven, it was the weekend and my husband was home; he came to the rescue. Later, he took me to the doctor and my head was still going round and round; it felt as though I was on a wild, spiraling ride through a dark tunnel with flashing lights. The diagnosis was an inner ear problem; a medication was prescribed that helped somewhat. However, for a long time when I would lay on my back and turn my head from side to side, the feeling of the wild ride would return and the ceiling would spin.

Bronchitis and colds seemed to come more frequently and stayed longer; I was given three or more shots of cortisone over a span of a year. Nothing else seemed to help this chronic condition which was worse in the fall of the year because of my allergy to ragweed.

In the spring of 1995, spongy, foul-smelling stools began to be a problem and my weight plummeted. Open bleeding sores appeared on my nose where my glasses rested. I saw a skin specialist who could not give an explanation for the occurrence. After that, an ophthalmologist thought maybe I had an allergy to the plastic nose pads on my eyeglasses and changed them. The sores remained, so I put small adhesive bandages on the spots.

Meanwhile, the spongy stools had become full blown diarrhea and my weight kept declining. My internist referred me to a gastroenterologist. When I met with the specialist several tests were scheduled for the following week. The results led him to the conclusion that I had a lactose intolerance. What a relief!

Immediately, all dairy products were excluded from my diet and I baked sourdough bread with water instead of milk, but matters only got worse. The diarrhea remained and became worse. It was constant and weight still rolled off, so I went back to the gastroenterologist. Another diagnosis was made ------SPRUE------(a.k.a. Celiac). He said, "Let's get you on a gluten-free diet." What was Sprue?? What was gluten?? The doctor sent me right over to the dietitian the same day. She explained the gluten-free diet and gave me a list of gluten-free foods. Wow, how simple? WRONG!!!

Shopping was a nightmare. It seemed that everything canned or processed had wheat, barley, or some other ingredient that was not allowed. The situation became overwhelming. Bread from the health food store made from rice flour tasted a bit worse than cardboard and had just about the same texture. More and more foods seemed to have gluten. My culinary world seemed to be getting smaller and smaller. Gluten was everywhere; like "the blob," it seemed to be covering everything in my path.

Trying to cope with the problem of obtaining gluten-free food was truly a challenge, but soon, after doing some research, my culinary world opened up once again. I changed my cooking habits to include more fresh vegetables in meals and prepared everything from scratch. This was quite a change from warming a frozen dinner in the microwave or fixing a box of something. I made a wise purchase, a bread machine. The freshly baked bread made from rice flour tasted like manna from heaven!

I had overcome one hurdle, gluten, but the bone and joint pain had not completely subsided and my back kept giving me fits. Sleep was still impossible; I would go from room to room at night dragging my pillow and blanket trying to find a comfortable spot. This was a nightly ritual.

A friend recommended a Florida clinic which specialized in back pain, so I decided to go since my children lived near the clinic. Staying with them while attending the clinic gave me the chance to play with my grandchildren.

The clinic set up appointments for three consecutive days. In the morning of the first day, I discussed my health history with the doctor who was quite knowledgeable about celiac disease. That afternoon I had some x-rays and nerve tests. Later in the evening, I had an MRI and in the last few minutes of the test an image enhancer was injected into my arm. Suddenly my ears started burning and itching and I asked the technicians if bugs were in their machine; they assured me there were no bugs anywhere. However, the tech noticed that my ears were very red; she stopped the test and helped me up. My legs started to tremble uncontrollably, then my arms. It looked like I was doing some strange new dance, but no music was playing and this was certainly not a party. The technicians decided to call someone else in the clinic who advised them to the notify the doctor on call. The doctor arrived promptly and quickly decided to order an ambulance to take me to a nearby emergency room. He mentioned, that to his knowledge, no one had ever had a reaction to the image enhancer that had been given to me.

The ambulance arrived shortly and the emergency medical technicians on board administered several IV's. When we arrived at the emergency room the doctor on duty gave me a shot of benadryl which eased the symptoms after a short time, but I was kept there for several hours just in case any more problems arose. It was nearly midnight before a call was placed to explain the situation to my son who had been quite worried because he had called the back clinic earlier, but no one answered. He came to pick me up because the doctor did not want me to drive after having a shot of benadryl. Finally, when we reached his house I fell into bed and slept for about 12 hours, the first good night's rest for me in years.

The second day I returned to the clinic and had a session of physical therapy. During a preliminary examination by the therapist, he noticed that my muscles seemed to be atrophied. I explained my diagnosis of celiac disease, then he concluded that the disorder caused this condition. My therapy included an hour of aquatic exercise which was very relaxing.

On the final day at the clinic the doctor discussed the results of my prior tests. The diagnosis of a degenerated spine and my knee problem was reconfirmed. Osteopenia, a precursor to osteoporosis, was suspected and a mild case of carpal tunnel syndrome was discovered. Hand splints were prescribed for the carpal tunnel; the doctor recommended that I start taking vitamin B-6 and have a bone density test and a bone scan after returning home. He referred me to a previous colleague who was now practicing at a clinic in Louisiana to monitor my back condition.

A few days after returning home I contacted the Louisiana clinic where I was scheduled to see a new doctor, an internist, who was to oversee my case. After going over my health history thoroughly, she was concerned that I was getting too little sleep. She prescribed a small dosage of Elavil for the problem, but the pill, she found out had starch in it. She kept searching her book and found that the liquid version contained NO GLUTEN. She ordered several blood tests for that same day.

The Elavil worked!! Sleep was like a wonder drug. The rest did me more good than anything else, because I started feeling much better.

The internist referred me to another doctor in the clinic. When we met, he reviewed my medical records and ordered a bone scan. The test was set up for the next week and the results were negative.

However, a bone density test was not as easy to schedule. It took about a month to see the doctor who had been recommended, but the time rolled by quickly. After I saw him it was another month before I had the test done and the results confirmed severe osteopenia. Fosamax, a bone building drug, calcium and vitamin D was prescribed.

After completing these tests I returned for another visit with the new internist who, after reviewing the results of prior tests, ordered more blood screening. The next day the phone rang and a nurse from the clinic in Louisiana said the results from those blood tests indicated that a particular substance in my blood was high and scheduled me an appointment for a short time later with two doctors of

133

oncology. When I saw them, they explained the situation and explained that the test results may indicate lymphoma which was quite a shock. Several weeks later a bone marrow biopsy was performed, a painful ordeal, but the results were negative. My blood still has to be monitored with regular tests every six months.

Because I had no problems it was several months before I made an appointment with the doctor who had been recommended to monitor my back. He reviewed my medical history and agreed with his colleague from Florida that exercise and physical therapy was the best approach for my pain.

After wearing splints on my hands and taking vitamin B-6 for several months the carpal tunnel subsided somewhat, but a slight tingling remained. Since the vitamin B-6 seemed to help I did more research about vitamin and some of my problems seemed to resemble symptoms of a vitamin deficiency. Who knows? But the idea of taking vitamins seemed sensible. My doctor agreed, but finding a gluten-free vitamin was quite a challenge. I learned a new fact: starch-free did not mean gluten-free, so I discontinued the vitamin B-6 because there was some question as to whether it was gluten-free even though it was starch-free. "The blob," gluten, kept getting in the way of my recuperation. Later, however, I located some gluten-free vitamins from the Solgar Company, who prints an easy to read booklet which provides information as to whether their products are gluten-free.

Finally, I discovered a local support group in a round about way when a friend, after hearing my story, mentioned that someone in her family also had celiac. Another friend who was present, later gave me a list of gluten-free foods which contained a contact number for CSA/USA. This was certainly a step in the right direction. Finding out that I did not stand alone was reassuring. Things were looking up.

What else could happen??? Female problems cropped up, so I made an appointment with my gynecologist. His recommendation was surgery, which was an extremely painful ordeal. I was given an epidural for anesthesia, but after the surgery it caused me to have a reaction of severe itching. The doctor ordered a shot, but it did not help. Soon the IV was terminated and the itching stopped. My back gave me a lot of trouble where the epidural was inserted. It was as if I had been cut at that spot with a machete, forcefully and the feeling remained for over a year.

A short time after the surgery, while bending over to pick up a tissue my back got stuck; I could not straighten up. Each time that I made a slight movement, my body rebelled with pain. After crawling to the bed I managed, somehow, to tumble into it which seemed to take forever. I called my husband who came to the rescue. The next day, after contacting the Louisiana clinic, he hauled me over ninety miles to see my back doctor. I had no appointment, but when I arrived the doctor saw me almost immediately. The diagnosis was soft tissue damage; a prescription for physical therapy and a pain medication was issued.

Later at physical therapy, my legs did not work very well and took a lot of determination just to turn the pedals of the stationary bike. However, the heat therapy and soft tissue massage helped tremendously. After about three weeks I noticed a slight improvement, but walking was still a chore.

Rest was not a problem anymore, but nonetheless, a very tired feeling began to settle into my body and nothing was interesting anymore. When I saw my internist, who suspected that I was depressed, she recommended a therapist. About a week later I saw a psychiatrist who listened to all my symptoms and the diagnosis of depression was confirmed. Even with all my personal and health problems, depression never seemed to bother me until now. You would think that somewhere in my past experiences depression would have surfaced, but this feeling was something new. I was given a prescription for a mild anti-depressant and regular weekly therapy sessions were scheduled with a psychologist. After a couple of months the depression began to lift and my interest in life started to return. Because my progress was positive the weekly sessions were replaced with monthly visits.

Recently, another bone density was performed and the results indicated that I had gained a significant amount of bone mass. Something seemed to be working, but then my short term memory started to fade; I stumbled over words frequently. Sometimes my tongue seemed like it was not connected to my brain. One particular occasion comes to mind, instead saying "days of the week," "days of the street came out." My mind seemed very fuzzy and my memory declined steadily. My internist, who thought maybe the symptoms indicated the early onset of Alzheimer's or a minor stroke, scheduled an MRI of my head. The results were negative. However, several doctors agreed, after further testing, that a definite problem existed, but slightly, and they concluded that being depressed was the root of my problems.

My therapy with the psychologist continued. She suggested that I initiate a project to fill my time. Since I had expanded my knowledge about celiac through research at the library and Internet sources, she said, "why don't you write a book about the disease, Aileen?" I thought this was an excellent idea.

Meanwhile, I had located a celiac newsgroup on the Internet which proved to be a another valuable source of information and after about a week of reading about all the problems that celiacs faced everyday, a light switched on in my head. The idea to write a book of true stories that illustrated how celiacs coped with their problems was initiated and the book project was launched. I decided that a part of the proceeds from this book would go to celiac research, which is truly needed in the U.S. Hopefully all my hours of poring over books, reading articles and surfing the Internet for information will help to educate the public to better understand the problems of celiacs.

The gluten-free diet has made quite a positive change in my life. My inner ear problem cleared up completely, the sores on my nose disappeared, my hair has regained its lost sheen, my skin is now moist, and a lot of my pain has ebbed, but my muscles are still weak.

Thanks to my husband, George, my book will come to fruition. Since sitting for a long period of time is still a problem for me, he does all the typing from my handwritten version. This has proven to be a task in itself, but we have survived and my appreciation to him cannot be expressed enough. Thanks again, George.

My culinary world has expanded greatly and I discover new dishes everyday. Some are quite delicious, but some are not. One cake turned out to be so hard after it was baked that I couldn't cut it; I pitched the whole thing out in the back yard for the birds, but they wouldn't touch it. The rain didn't even melt it, so finally, I tossed it in the garbage. Here is a better recipe that I will share with you

BAKED TOMATOES WITH CORNBREAD CRUMBS

2 or 3 tomatoes--sliced about 1 inch thick
Olive oil
1 or 2 Purple onions--sliced
Oregano
Basil
Salt and pepper
Left over cornbread--make into crumbs--about a cupful
Garlic--about 1 teaspoon minced
Grated cheddar or mozzarella cheese--about a cup

Place the sliced tomatoes in a greased Pyrex dish or

baking pan. 11 3/4 x 7 1/2 x 3/4

Drizzle the tomato with olive oil and sprinkle with oregano, basil, salt and pepper--as much or as little as you prefer. Then put some grated cheese. Place a slice of onion on top of cheese--drizzle the onion with oil and sprinkle with spices, then add more cheese

Brown the cornbread crumbs with garlic on medium heat (about 5 minutes or so) and sprinkle them on top of tomato-onion-cheese pile. Cook in a 350 degree oven until the tomatoes and onions are cooked--about 30 minutes.

This recipe is great because you don't have to measure, just pile everything up like a sandwich and bake. Cornbread crumbs are delicious and crunchy; however, you can substitute any kind of crumbs that you wish, just whatever is handy. This is my kind of cooking-easy, flexible and quick!!

REMARKS

The stories reflect several things, but most of all they demonstrate that celiac disease is sometimes difficult to diagnose. Each case had a unique set of symptoms; some had no visible symptoms with the onset occurring at different times. This uniqueness seems to be a common thread that weaves through all celiacs' lives, binding each different case into a tapestry of symptoms that change from individual to individual like a chameleon that changes color with his background which makes the diagnosis difficult. The stories certainly have demonstrated that celiac disease is a "great masquerader."

In some cases symptoms went dormant, yet in other cases they only escalated. One mystery that remains unsolved: why does celiac go dormant? Maybe the answer will be uncovered in the future by research.

Heritage plays a big part in the disease and how it affects our lives. The ties that we share in our dietary world seem to make us the celiac clan, one big family with members all over the world; no matter where you meet a celiac you share an instant bond.

The stories illustrated, in some cases, a vitamin deficiency existed. Included in the next chapter is a short reference about vitamins, compliments of Solgar Vitamin and Herb Company. This information will help you to be informed, so that you can ask your doctor more prudent questions. Before starting any regimen of vitamins or supplements you should seek the advice of your physician and continued use should be closely monitored by your physician.

VITAMIN	U.S. RDA*	BIOLOGICAL FUNCTION
VITAMIN A/ BETA CAROTENE	**5000 IU**	Maintenance of healthy skin, eyes, bones, hair and teeth. Beta Carotene is an an antioxidant and can be converted by the body to Vitamin A as needed.
VITAMIN D	**400 IU**	Assists in the absorption and metabolism of calcium and phosphorus for strong bones and teeth.
VITAMIN E	**30 IU**	As an antioxidant, helps protect cell membranes, lipoprotiens, fats and Vitamin A from destructive oxidation. Helps protect red blood cells.
VITAMIN K	******	Needed for proper blood clotting.

VITAMIN	U.S. RDA *	BIOLOGICAL FUNCTION
VITAMIN C	**60 mg**	As antioxidant, inhibits the formation of nitrosamines (a suspected carcinogen). Important for maintenance of bones, teeth, collagen and blood vessels (capillaries). Enhances iron absorption, red blood formation.
VITAMIN B-1 (Thiamin)	**1.5 mg**	Releases energy from foods. Needed for normal appetite and for functioning of nervous system.
VITAMIN B-2 (Riboflavin)	**1.7 mg**	Releases energy from foods. Necessary for healthy skin and eyes.
VITAMIN B-3 (Niacin)	**20 mg**	Releases energy from foods. Aids in maintenance of skin, nervous system, and proper mental functioning.
VITAMIN B-6 (Pyridoxine)	**2 mg**	Releases energy from foods. Plays a role in protein and fat metabolism. Essential for function of red blood cells and hemoglobin synthesis.

VITAMIN	U.S. RDA *	BIOLOGICAL FUNCTION
VITAMIN B-12	**6 mcg**	Prevents pernicious anemia. Necessary for a healthy nervous system. Involved in synthesis of genetic material. (DNA)
BIOTIN	**300 mcg**	Releases energy from foods. Plays a role in metabolism of amino acids. Needed for normal hair production and growth.
PANTOTHENIC ACID	**10 mg**	Releases energy from foods. Involved in synthesis of acetylcholine, an excitatory neurotransmitter. Needed for normal function of the adrenal glands.
FOLIC ACID	**400 mcg**	Necessary for proper red blood cell formation. Plays a role in the metabolism of fats, amino acids, DNA and RNA. Needed for proper cell division and protein synthesis.

VITAMINS   U.S. RDA * BIOLOGICAL FUNCTION

CHOLINE ~   ******   As a lipotropic nutrient, prevents fat accumulation in the liver. Precursor to acetycholine, a major neurotransmitter to the brain.

INSITOL   ******   Involved in calcium mobilization.

\\\

MINERALS   U.S. RDA* BIOLOGICAL FUNCTION

BORON~   ******   Possibly plays a role in maintaining strong bones. Affects calcium and magnesium metabolism. May be needed for proper membrane function.

CALCIUM   **1000 mg**   Builds strong bones and teeth. Involved in nerve transmission and muscle contraction.

144

MINERALS   U.S. RDA* BIOLOGICAL FUNCTION

CHROMIUM   **   A part of Glucose
Tolerance Factor (GTF),
it works with insulin to
regulate blood sugar levels.

COPPER   **2 mg**   Essential for red blood
cell formation, and
hemoglobin synthesis.
Involved in many
enzyme systems
including, superoxide
dismutase (SOD), a
major antioxidant
enzyme system.

IODINE   **150 mcg**   Needed for proper
functioning of the thyroid
gland and production of
thyroid hormones.

IRON   **18 mg**   Prevents anemia; as a
constituent of
hemoglobin, transports
oxygen throughout the
body.

MAGNESIUM   **400 mg**   Needed in many enzyme
systems, especially those
involved with energy
production. Essential for
heartbeat and nerve
transmission. Constituent
of bones and teeth.

MINERALS   U.S. RDA*   BIOLOGICAL FUNCTION

MANGANESE   **   Cofactor in many enzyme
                             systems including those
                             involved in bone
                             formation, energy
                             production and protein
                             metabolism.

MOLYBDENUM   **   Required for proper
                             growth and development.
                             Plays a role in fat and
                             nucleic acid metabolism.
                             Needed for proper
                             sulfur metabolism.

PHOSPHORUS   1000 mg   Maintains strong bones
                             and teeth. Necessary
                             for muscle and nerve
                             function.

POTASSIUM   **   An electrolyte needed
                             to maintain fluid balance,
                             proper heartbeat and
                             nerve transmission.

SELENIUM   **   As an antioxidant, it is
                             a constituent of
                             glutathione peroxidase.
                             Protects vitamin E.

SILICON~   **   Needed for proper
                             bone structure and growth.

MINERALS U.S. RDA* BIOLOGICAL FUNCTION

ZINC   15 mg   Component of insulin;
                                        required for blood sugar
                                        control. Needed for
                                        proper taste and hearing.
                                        Important in wound
                                        healing and enzyme
                                        activation.

* U.S. RDA=United States recommend daily allowance as
established by the Federal Food and Drug Administration
** No U.S. RDA has been established.
~Nutrients essential for some higher animals but not proven
to be necessary for humans.

3. From: Solgar Vitamin and Herb Company
         500 Willow Tree Road
         Leonia, NJ 07605
         Permission given by Paul Zullo
         www.solgar.com
         feedback@solgar.com
         201-944-2311   FAX 201-944-7351

GLOSSARY

AMENORRHEA--An abnormal stoppage or absence of the menstrual flow.

APHTHOUS STOMATIS--Inflammation of the oral membrane, which may involve the entire mouth.

ANEMIA--A condition in which the blood is deficient in quantity or quality. The deficiency in quality may consist of a diminished amount of hemoglobin or in a diminished number of red blood corpuscles, or both.

ANTIBODY--A substance that attaches to cells and sensitizes the cells or render them susceptible to destruction by body defenses.

ANTIGEN--A substance or organism, when foreign to the blood stream, upon gaining access to the tissues, stimulates the formation of a specific antibody and reacts specifically to neutralize or destroy it.

ASYMPTOMATIC--Showing or causing no symptoms.

BIOPSY--Removal and examination, usually microscopic, of tissue or other material from the living body for purposes of diagnosis.

CRYPT--A minute tubelike depression opening on a free surface.

DERMATITIS HERPETIFORMIS--An inflammation of the skin marked by clusters of blisters accompanied by burning and itching.

EDEMA--The presence of abnormally large amounts of fluid in the intercellular tissue spaces of the body.

ENTERITIS--Inflammation of the intestines, chiefly of the small intestines.

ETIOLOGY--The study or theory of the causation of any diseases. adj. **etiologic.**

FOLATE--One of the B-complex vitamins.

GLIADIN--An alcohol-soluble protein obtainable from wheat.

GLOBIN--Protein constituent of the *hemoglobin*.

GLUTEN--Protein found in wheat and other grains which gives the dough its tough elastic characteristics.

HEMATINIC--A substance which is effective in increasing the oxygen content of the blood and increasing the number of red corpuscles.

HEMAGLOBIN--The oxygen-carrying red pigment of the red corpuscles.

HISTOLOGY--Science of tissues, including their cellular composition and organization. (adj. Histologic)

HYPOPROTEINEMIA--Abnormal decrease in the amount of protein in the blood.

JEJUNUM--That portion of the small intestine which extends from the duodenum (first part of the intestine) and the ileum (beginning of the large intestine).

LYMPHOCYTE--A variety of white blood corpuscles which arises in the reticular tissue of the lymph glands.

LYMPHOMA--Any tumor, made up of the lymphoid tissue.

MUCOSA--A thin layer of tissue which covers a surface or divides a space or organ. Mucous membrane.

PARESTHESIA--An abnormal sensation such as tingling, burning, or prickling.

PROGNOSIS--A forecast to the probable result of an attack of disease. The prospect as to the recovery from a disease as indicated by the nature and symptoms of the case.

QUERULOUS--Full of complaint, peevish, cranky.

REFRACTOY--Not readily yielding to treatment.

STEATORRHEA--The presence of excess fat in the stool.

SYMPTOM---Any functional evidence of disease or of a patient's condition; a change in a patients condition.

VILLUS--Threadlike projections covering the mucosa in the small intestine.

2. From <u>Dorland's Illustrated Medical Dictionary,</u> Twenty-third Edition, Editorial Board, Leslie Brainerd Arey, Ph.D., Sc.D., LL.D.; Robert Laughlin Rea Professor of Anatomy, Northwestern University; William Burrows, Ph.D., Professor of Microbology, The University of Chicago; J.P. Greenhill, MD, Professor of Gynecology, Cook County Graduate School of Medicine; Richard M. Hewitt, A.M., MD, Senior Consultant, Section of Publications, The Mayo Clinic.

Philadelphia:W. B. Saunders Company-1957

1. From: <u>The Merck Manual of Diagnosis and</u>
        <u>Therapy,</u> Edition 16,
        pp.826-828.
        Edited by Robert Berkow
        Rahway, NJ: Merck & Co., Inc.,1992

2. From: <u>Dorland's Illustrated Medical Dictionary</u>
        Twenty-Third Edition
        Editorial Board, Leslie Brainerd Arey,
        Ph.D., Sc.D., LL.D; Robert Laughlin Rea,
        Professor of Anatomy, Northwestern
        University; William Burrows, Ph.D.
        Professor of Microbiology, The University
        of Chicago; J.P. Greenhill, M.D.,
        Professor of Gynecology, Cook County
        Graduate School of Medicine;
        Richard M. Hewitt, A.M.,M.D., Senior
        Consultant, Section of Publications
        The Mayo Clinic.
        Philadelphia: W.B.Saunders
        Company-1957

3.. From: <u>A Guide to Vitamins and Minerals</u>
        Solgar Vitamin and Herb Company
        500 Willow Tree Road
        Leonia, NJ 07605
        Permission given by Paul Zullo
        www.solgar.com
        feedback@solgar.com
        201-944-2311
        201-944-7351 Fax

COPING WITH CELIAC
ORDER FORM

U.S.Price.......$12.99..... add shipping and handling....$4.00

Shipping and handling: Canada, Ireland, England...$5.00

Other shipping $6.00 or more

U.S.Dollars only

Ship To:

Name:..

Address..

Postal

.............................Code.................Country..............

Bill To:

Master/Visa Card

Number..

Expiration Date..

If billing name is different from shipping name, enter:

Name..

Address..

Postal

.............................Code.................Country..............

FOR FASTER SERVICE CALL

1-877-896-9334 (Toll free U.S.only)

OR

SEND CHECK

All checks must be made out in U.S. Dollars only

TO:

A & G PUBLISHING

2907 PALMER DR.

GULFPORT, MS   39507

Please include proper shipping charges